The Metabolic Maze

Copyright © 2023 Joshua Bassett

All rights reserved.

ISBN: 9798865689171

Joshua Bassett is a personal trainer who is looking to pursue a degree in nutrition. He has studied anatomy, nutrition, physiology, and sport psychology, for which he holds a recognized national diploma.

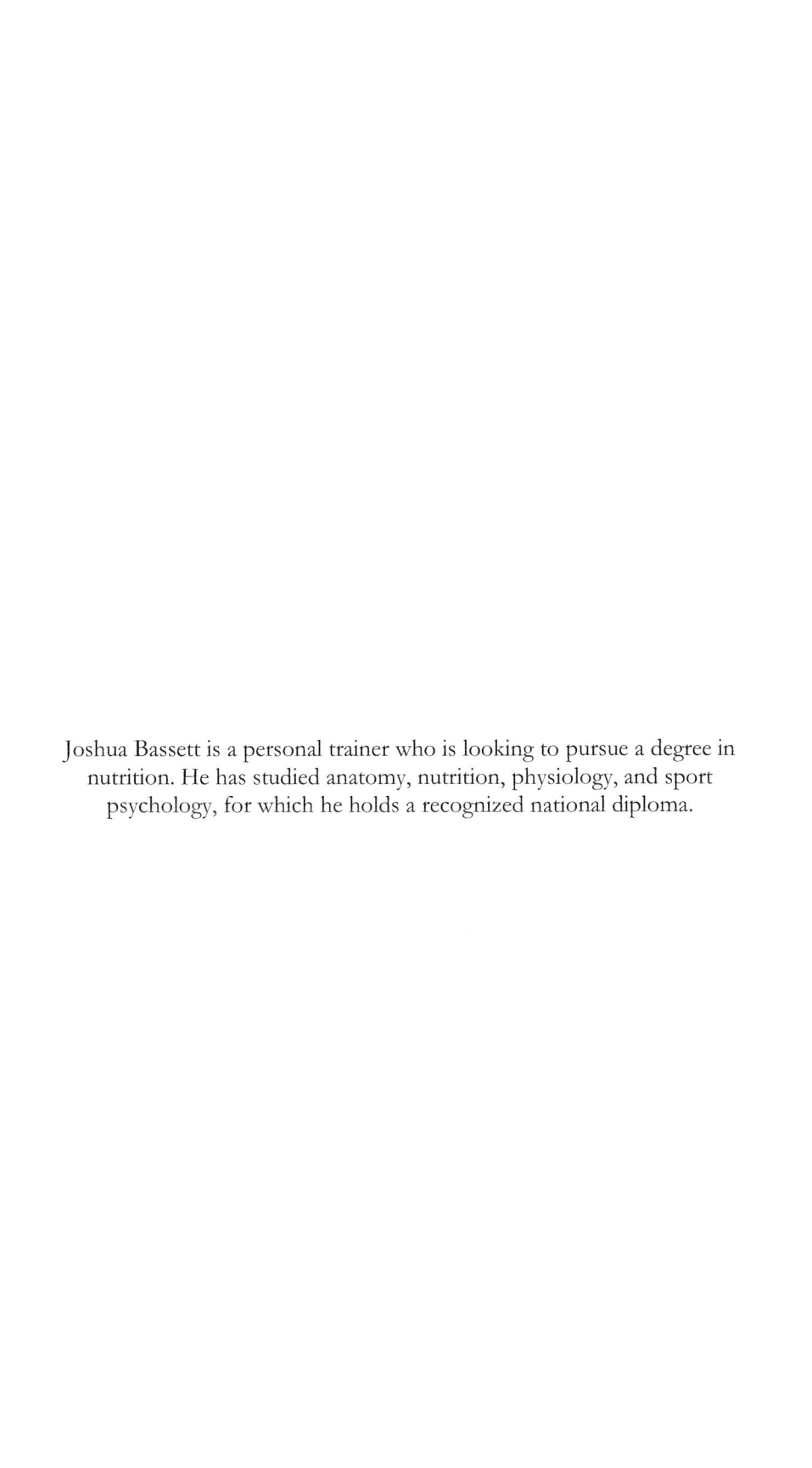

CONTENTS

Acknowledgments

Personal Note

1	Detoxify or not	2
2	Understanding the problem	5
3	Revealing invisible health risks	34
4	Read your labels	58
	Non-toxic grocery list	57
5	The fitness puzzle	64
6	The road to relief	71
7	Personal Care Products	106

ACKNOWLEDGMENTS

This book was designed and published by Joshua Bassett. For all resources you can contact joshbassetfit@gmail.com or go to www.joshbassettfitness.com.

MEDICAL DISCLAIMER

The information provided in this book is for informational and educational purposes only. It is not intended as a substitute for professional medical advice, diagnosis, or treatment. Always seek the advice of your physician or other qualified health provider with any questions you may have regarding a medical condition.

The author of this book is not a medical professional, and the content presented here should not be considered as medical advice. Any information or guidance provided in this book should not be used to diagnose, treat, cure, or prevent any medical condition.

It is essential to consult with a qualified healthcare provider before making any significant decisions about your health, including starting or discontinuing any course of treatment, changing your medication, or adopting any specific lifestyle changes.

The author and publisher do not assume any responsibility for any potential consequences resulting from the use of the information contained in this book. You are solely responsible for your health and well-being, and any decisions you make should be made in consultation with a healthcare professional.

PERSONAL NOTE

My name is Joshua Bassett, and I'm not here to impress you with fancy titles or lofty credentials. Instead, I am on a winding path towards health and well-being, seeking answers and sharing discoveries that have shaped my perspective. My journey has been marked by personal challenges, including battles with arthritis and psoriasis, but it has also been profoundly influenced by the health struggles of those dearest to me.

My mother's diagnosis of rheumatoid arthritis and lymphedema, the persistent trials faced by family members grappling with IBS, and the presence of metabolic diseases in our circle of friends have fuelled my quest for understanding. Over the past four years, I've embarked on a relentless pursuit of knowledge, immersing myself in research that delves deep into the intersections of nutrition, fitness, and health.

What has emerged from my research is a realization that health is not a passive state but an active choice. The decisions we make about what we consume and how we live exert a profound influence on our well-being. In the pages ahead, I invite you to join me as we explore the intricate relationship between our dietary choices, lifestyle, and how health has changed among humans in the previous decades.

While we'll certainly uncover some unsettling truths about foods that are considered nutritious, this journey is not about fearmongering. It's a call to action, an opportunity to make informed decisions that empower us to reclaim control over our health. So, let's embark on this journey together as we unveil the facts about our food, share non-toxic recipes, and forge a path towards a brighter, healthier future—one step, one bite at a time.

DETOXIFY OR NOT

In a world that is devaluing health and wellness, it's not unusual for individuals to make assumptions about their own well-being. Many people equate feeling good or the absence of obvious symptoms with being healthy. They might think, "I eat well enough," "I exercise occasionally," or "I don't feel sick, so I must be healthy." However, these assumptions can create a false sense of security.

The reality is that health is a multifaceted concept that goes beyond the mere absence of symptoms. It encompasses a complex interplay of physical, mental, and emotional factors. While feeling well is certainly a positive indicator, it doesn't always provide a comprehensive picture of one's overall health. In fact, underlying health issues can silently develop over time, often going unnoticed.

Our modern lifestyles expose us to potential health risks, ranging from environmental toxins to stress-inducing factors. These hidden dangers can accumulate within our bodies, gradually impacting our well-being without our awareness. Therefore, it's crucial to move beyond assumptions and take concrete steps to assess and address our health.

Think of the tip of the iceberg as what we can readily see—our external well-being. It's the visible part above the waterline. However, most of the iceberg lies beneath the surface, concealed from view. This concealed portion symbolises the intricacy of our health, encompassing factors such as nutrition, environmental exposures, stress levels, and more.

To determine the approximate levels of toxicity in your body and gain a more accurate understanding of your health, consider the following self-assessment. This tool can help you recognize potential areas of concern and guide you toward a more informed approach to well-being.

Instructions: Please check the boxes next to the statements that apply to your current situation or experience. Be honest with your responses to get an accurate assessment of your potential need for a potential change.

☐ I often consume processed and fast foods.

☐ My diet is high in sugar and unhealthy fats.

☐ I frequently experience digestive issues like bloating or gas.

☐ I have chronic skin problems (e.g., acne, eczema).

☐ My sleep quality is poor, and I often feel restless.

☐ I experience mood swings, anxiety, or depression regularly.

☐ Maintaining a healthy weight has been challenging for me.

☐ I am currently taking medications for chronic health issues.

☐ I often feel stressed and have difficulty managing it.

☐ I consume alcohol and caffeine frequently.

☐ I engage in regular physical activity or exercise rarely or never.

☐ I often forget to drink enough water throughout the day.

☐ I have known allergies or food sensitivities.

☐ I am regularly exposed to environmental toxins (e.g., pollution, chemicals).

☐ I have dental issues or frequent dental problems.

☐ I experience frequent common illnesses like colds or infections.

☐ I consume highly processed or fast foods frequently.

☐ I deal with chronic pain or discomfort.

☐ I have experienced adverse reactions to specific foods (e.g., hives, digestive issues).

☐ My overall sense of well-being is currently poor.

Scoring:

0-5 Checked Statements: Low Toxicity Level

6-10 Checked Statements: Moderate Toxicity Level

11-15 Checked Statements: High Toxicity Level

16-20 Checked Statements: Very High Toxicity Level

After completing this self-assessment, you'll have a better sense of potential areas where your health may need attention. This is just the beginning of your journey to optimal well-being. Understanding your health is the first step towards making informed choices and positive changes.

UNDERSTANDING THE PROBLEM

The modern world presents us with an evolving health landscape characterised by complex challenges. Chronic diseases, autoimmune conditions, and reproductive health problems are on the rise, affecting millions worldwide. We begin our journey by examining the data, insights from medical literature, and personal stories that underscore the urgency of addressing these issues.

To navigate this metabolic maze, we must dive deep into the possible triggers behind these health challenges. This exploration has led us to factors such as changes in lifestyle, dietary habits and environmental influences. By understanding the "why" behind these issues, you will be better equipped to make informed decisions about your health.

The quest is not limited to individual experiences; it extends to a global perspective. These health challenges transcend around the world, affecting individuals from diverse backgrounds. By recognising the universality of these concerns, you may discover a greater connection with people worldwide facing similar health issues.

As we embark on this journey together, keep in mind that your health is a valuable treasure. With knowledge as our guide, we will navigate the metabolic maze, uncover hidden truths, and embark on a path toward enhanced health, vitality, and balance. So, let's begin and explore the complexities of health in the modern world.

Diabetes is a widespread condition which has emerged as a significant health concern, affecting millions of lives worldwide. As we delve deeper into the data, personal stories, and medical insights, we shed light on the urgency of addressing this growing crisis.

Diabetes is not just a disease; it's a global health crisis. Its prevalence has surged, and its impact on individuals and communities is profound. Through compelling data and real-life narratives, I aim to provide a comprehensive view of the diabetes epidemic's scale and scope.

Quoted by The World Health Organization "In 2014, 8.5% of adults aged 18 years and older had diabetes. In 2019, diabetes was the direct cause of 1.5 million deaths and 48% of all deaths due to diabetes occurred before the age of 70 years.

Another 460 000 kidney disease deaths were caused by diabetes, and raised blood glucose causes around 20% of cardiovascular deaths (1).

Between 2000 and 2019, there was a 3% increase in age-standardized mortality rates from diabetes. In lower-middle-income countries, the mortality rate due to diabetes increased 13%."

Over the course of time, diabetes can lead to the deterioration of blood vessels in vital organs such as the heart, eyes, kidneys, and nerves. Individuals living with diabetes face an elevated risk of various health complications, including but not limited to heart attacks, strokes, and kidney dysfunction. Diabetes has the potential to result in irreversible vision impairment by impairing the blood vessels within the eyes. Type 1 diabetes (T1D) is an autoimmune disease where the body's immune system mistakenly attacks and destroys insulin-producing cells in the pancreas. It's influenced by both genetics and environmental factors. However, even identical twins may not both develop the disease, suggesting that environmental factors also play a role.

Environmental factors can affect how our genes work, even though they don't change the genes themselves. In the case of Type 1 Diabetes (T1D), these effects, called epigenetic changes, can lead to genes not working correctly. These changes happen through processes like DNA methylation, histone modifications, and miRNA regulation. In simple terms, it's how our environment can impact our genes and contribute to T1D.

These epigenetic changes impact genes related to antigen presentation, immune tolerance, the response of autoreactive T cells, and the function of insulin-producing cells. Your risk of developing type 2 diabetes is higher if you lead a sedentary lifestyle, carry excess weight or being obese. Being overweight can lead to insulin resistance, a common factor in type 2 diabetes. Certain hormonal disorders can be the cause as well such as Excessive cortisol production, an overproduction- on of human growth hormone, as-well as hyperthyroidism.

Pancreatitis, pancreatic cancer, or a trauma injury can damage beta cells, reducing the ability to produce insulin, which can lead to diabetes. If the pancreas is surgically removed, diabetes may develop due to the loss of these beta cells. Gestational diabetes mellitus (GDM) is defined as any level of glucose intolerance that begins or is first identified during pregnancy.

Many clinical factors have been identified as potential risk factors for developing gestational diabetes. These factors include having an elevated body weight, leading a less active lifestyle, or giving birth to a new-born with macrosomia and metabolic comorbidities like hypertension.

Low levels of HDL cholesterol, triglyceride levels greater than 250, the presence of polycystic ovarian syndrome, haemoglobin A1C levels exceeding 5.7, abnormal results from an oral glucose tolerance test, any significant indicator of insulin resistance (such as acanthosis nigricans), and a past medical history of cardiovascular diseases also contribute to the risk profile for gestational diabetes.

Now that we know what diabetes is, what has changed over the years for this to become a massive problem?

Industrial seed oils, much like refined sugar and excess calories, present a disconnect from our evolutionary history. Prior to the 1900s, industrial seed oils were not a part of the human diet. However, between 1970 and 2000, the average yearly consumption of one such oil like soybean oil, surged from four pounds per person to 26 pounds per person!

In today's diet, linoleic acid, the primary fatty acid found in industrial seed oils, makes up 8 percent of our total calorie intake. In contrast, our hunter-gatherer ancestors consumed only 1 to 3 percent of their total calories in the form of linoleic acid.

Experts are very knowledgeable about the concept of evolutionary mismatch propose that our bodies are not designed to cope with such a substantial intake of linoleic acid. Consequently, our elevated consumption of industrial seed oils is having detrimental effects on our health.

The polyunsaturated fatty acids found in industrial seed oils are highly susceptible to oxidisation when exposed to factors like heat, light, and certain chemicals. This leads to the formation of two harmful substances: trans fats and lipid peroxides.

Trans fats are widely recognized for their detrimental impact on health, contributing to the development of cardiovascular disease and type 2 diabetes. In fact, for every 2 percent increase in calories derived from trans fats, the risk of heart disease nearly doubles.

On the other hand, lipid peroxides are toxic by-products that inflict damage on DNA, proteins, and cell membrane lipids throughout the body. The accumulation of lipid peroxides in the body is associated with accelerated aging and the onset of chronic diseases.

Next time you fill your cap up, go to your local shop and stick some canola oil in there. It should run smooth.

Apart from STAYING CLEAR of seed oils and considering genetic predispositions, based on my perspective as a personal trainer with over six years of experience, here are some recommendations to lower your risk of developing diabetes.

Keep your weight under control, using a BMI calculator as your method of use is inaccurate as you may have high amounts of muscle at 8% body and be considered fat or obese. It is far easier to take your shirt off, look in the mirror and be honest with yourself.

Now how can we keep our weight under control? Cardiovascular exercise is one big preventative method as moving more than 30 minutes a day 5 days a week will reduce chances as this will enable the muscle cells to use insulin and glucose more efficiently.

Strength training is very important, the less muscle mass you have, the less your lymphatic fluid moves. This means you have a higher risk of high triglycerides, high cholesterol and to inability remove toxic waste from your body. I'm not saying go crazy and deadlift crazy amounts of weight. All you must do is contract your muscle with a full range of motion whilst under tension. So, if you have 30 minutes a day to exercise, go the gym.

Chronic stress can contribute to the development of diabetes due to excess cortisol levels. Incorporate stress-reduction techniques into your daily routine, such as deep breathing exercises, yoga, or spending time in nature. Managing stress effectively can help regulate blood sugar levels and reduce the risk of diabetes.

Based on current scientific insights, it is widely believed that weight loss plays a pivotal role in achieving remission in type 2 diabetes. According to a prominent theory known, the accumulation of excess fat in the liver, brought about by weight gain, leads to the storage of fat within the pancreas. This, in turn, hinders the proper functioning of insulin-producing beta cells. Many doctors and scientists believe that by losing overall body weight, individuals can reduce fat accumulation within the pancreas, thereby facilitating the restoration of normal insulin production.

Regardless of how one defines remission, it's important to recognize that any reduction in A1C levels and/or successful weight loss can significantly diminish the risk of enduring long-term complications.

Beyond health benefits, achieving remission brings with it several other compelling advantages. This encompasses an enhanced sense of well-being, and the liberation from ongoing medication use.

While it's crucial to understand that discontinuing all medications may not be the ultimate objective for individuals with diabetes, particularly considering the advances in heart and kidney protection offered by drugs like GLP-1 agonists and SGLT-2 inhibitors, reducing reliance on one or more medications can lead to fewer side effects and notable financial savings.

However, it is important to understand that diabetes represents just one piece of a puzzle within metabolic maze. As you turn the pages, you will find links and the same if not similar potential causes of these diseases.

Autoimmune diseases, over 80 in number and counting, collectively represent a vast and complex landscape. From the well-known diseases like rheumatoid arthritis and multiple sclerosis to the lesser known as Grave's disease, yet equally formidable conditions which affect millions of lives worldwide. Their symptoms are as diverse as their names, spanning from joint pain and fatigue to neurological impairments and skin rashes.

But it's not just their diversity that scares me; it's the intricate interplay of genes, environment, and autoimmune responses to food that gives rise to these complex disorders. How does a person's own immune system become a traitor? What prompts it to attack the very body it is meant to protect? These are the questions that continue to baffle researchers and medical professionals.

T cells, play a pivotal role in our immune system by employing specialized receptors on their surfaces to discern foreign bacteria's and viruses. Ordinarily, T cells that react against our own bodily tissues undergo elimination by the thymus, a crucial immune organ situated behind the breastbone.

However, occasionally, a fraction of these self-reactive T cells evades this elimination process. They can become activated through mechanisms that are not yet fully understood, potentially involving factors such as viral infections or hormonal cues. Once activated, these renegade T cells assume the role of commanders, issuing instructions to B cells, prompting them to generate antibodies targeted at specific components of our body, such as tissues or organs. This process creates an autoimmune response, where your body starts attacking itself.

Rheumatoid arthritis is inflammation or swelling in one or more joints. This is a persistent inflammatory condition, often resulting from the interplay of genetic factors combined with food and environmental triggers like the inhalation of tobacco. It primarily affects the synovial joints. Typically, it initiates in smaller peripheral joints, exhibiting a symmetric pattern, and, if not managed, extends to impact proximal joints. Prolonged joint inflammation will lead to joint deterioration, involving cartilage loss and bone erosion.

Now, as much as I would like to write about all the arthritis types which accounts for over one hundred different types, there is not enough evidence and research about them all which is why I have chosen RA. I also have a lot of experience with this specific condition of arthritis as a personal trainer and someone who lives in the same household with a sufferer.

Diagnosing rheumatoid arthritis in its early stages can be challenging because there isn't a pathognomonic lab test that can confirm it. To accurately identify this condition and prevent severe joint damage, a thorough clinical evaluation is necessary by a rheumatologist. Managing patients with rheumatoid arthritis involves a combination of medications and non-pharmacological approaches.

My journey as a personal trainer has revealed the resilience and determination of individuals battling rheumatoid arthritis. It has been a humbling experience to witness the strength and commitment of my clients and family as they strive to maintain their physical well-being amidst the challenges posed by RA.

The blood tests aim to detect inflammation and specific blood proteins (antibodies) associated with RA:

Erythrocyte sedimentation rate (ESR, commonly referred to as "sed rate") and C-reactive protein (CRP) levels serve as indicators of inflammation. When elevated ESR or CRP levels are coupled with other RA-related indicators, they contribute to the diagnostic process. Although you can have high CRP markers without having RA. Rheumatoid factor (RF) is an antibody detected in approximately 80 percent of individuals with RA, albeit not immediately. Antibodies targeting cyclic citrullinated peptide

(CCP) are present in around 60 to 70 percent of RA cases. It's important to note that CCP antibodies can also be present in individuals who do not have RA.

The objectives in the management of rheumatoid arthritis (RA) are wide and takes hard work.

First and foremost, the primary aim is to reduce inflammation, ideally achieving a state of remission where the disease's activity is subdued. This entails significantly reducing the inflammatory processes within the body.

In addition to reducing inflammation, another critical goal is to alleviate the often-debilitating symptoms that accompany RA, such as joint pain, swelling, and stiffness. Improving your quality of life by providing relief from these distressing symptoms is an integral part of RA treatment.

Osteoarthritis cases have surged by 449% since the 1990s. RA cases have increased by 36.30% since 2004. So, what is causing these inflammatory responses. What is the elusive trigger behind the relentless inflammatory responses in arthritis, a question that has perplexed scientists and researchers for decades? Is it a complex interplay of genetic predisposition and environmental factors, or is there a hidden culprit lurking within our immune system? Are there specific dietary choices that play a role, or perhaps infectious agents that go unnoticed?

Accumulating research findings indicate that nutrition may play a role in both the onset and the management of rheumatoid arthritis (RA).

There are many ways to reduce inflammatory with anti-inflammatory diets known as the Mediterranean diet, FODMAP, elemental dieting, animal-based dieting and DASH dieting. For me personally and what I have learned from experience is that the animal-based diet works for me, and the Mediterranean diet works best for others.

Navigating inflammatory responses and arthritis often entails a process of diligent elimination and discovery. Much like a detective on a mission, individuals may need to exclude certain foods or dietary components to identify triggers of inflammation that are unique to their bodies through a process of elimination. This process can be a transformative journey, one that necessitates patience, and a keen awareness of how different foods impact your personal well-being and inflammatory responses.

Bowel irritability is on the rise, and it can be aggressive. There are four different syndrome subcategories (IBS) and 2 main chronic diseases (IBD).

Irritable Bowel Syndrome (IBS), a functional gastrointestinal disorder that implies a disturbance in the normal functioning of the bowels. The impact of IBS on an individual's well-being is profound, ranging from mild discomfort to debilitating symptoms that significantly affect their self-perception.

Furthermore, individuals diagnosed with IBS often have a higher likelihood of experiencing other functional disorders such as fibromyalgia, chronic fatigue syndrome, chronic pelvic pain, or temporomandibular joint disorder (TMJ). IBS is prevalent, affecting at least 10 to 15 percent of adults in the United States, with a higher incidence in women than in men.

IBD is an acronym for inflammatory bowel disease, a term used to encompass conditions characterized by persistent inflammation within the gastrointestinal (GI) tract. The two main forms of IBD include Crohn's disease and ulcerative colitis.

Crohn's disease causes inflammation in the digestive tract, causing symptoms such as abdominal pain, diarrhoea, fatigue, weight loss, and malnutrition. The inflammation associated with Crohn's disease may affect segments of the digestive tract, with the small intestine being the most frequently inflamed, although this varies from person to person.

Ulcerative colitis is a persistent condition characterized by inflammation in the colon and rectum. This inflammation can cause small ulcers on the lining of the colon, which may result in bleeding and pus.

What are the mysterious components lurking within our daily sustenance that can send our digestive systems into disarray? Is it the preservatives, the additives, or the unpronounceable ingredients that we've come to accept as commonplace in our meals? Could it be the imbalance between processed and natural foods, or perhaps the relentless pursuit of convenience over nutrition? And why does it appear that IBS and other gastrointestinal disorders are on the rise with our evolving dietary habits? These questions compel us to delve deep into the heart of our modern food culture, to scrutinize the choices we make at the grocery store and the impact they have on our digestive well-being.

After thorough research, there is an outstanding amount of misleading research into the treatment of Crohn's disease. Unlike the FODMAP diet using to help treat IBS. There is no cure for Crohn's disease, which means the closest thing you are going to get to a cure is diet.

Human studies have shown that an imbalanced ratio between omega -6 and omega-3 fatty acids are highly correlated. These results indicate that a diet rich in omega-6 fatty acids can modify the composition of the gut microbiota, creating an inflammatory response in the gastrointestinal tract, potentially playing a role in the onset of conditions like IBS and IBD. This is all done through the consumption industrial seed oils.

Sucralose may have a detrimental impact on individuals with inflammatory bowel disease (IBD). The evidence indicates that Sucralose could potentially exacerbate IBD-related conditions by intensifying inflammation within the gastrointestinal tract. Everyone i know and from personal experience who eats nightshades and certain cruciferous vegetables suffer badly from abdominal pain, bloating, nausea and in some cases diarrhoea. As you turn pages, you will find more information about these certain plants containing defence chemicals inside them which cause inflammatory responses and in some cases poisoning. Nightshades share a defence chemical known as glycoalkaloids. Studies have shown that the glycoalkaloid concentration in potatoes have been proven to adversely affect the small intestine, which aggravates IBD.

Lectins, classified as proteins with an affinity for carbohydrates, serve as protective agents for plants in nature. However, when it comes to human digestion, the very characteristics that make lectins defence mechanisms, could lead to complications. Lectins have the capacity to attach themselves to the cells that line the digestive tract, potentially interfering with the breakdown and absorption of nutrients, as well as influencing the development and behaviour of intestinal flora. Given their prolonged binding to cells, lectin proteins could trigger autoimmune responses within your gut.

In conclusion, it is evident that certain plants, additives and industrial seed oils contain chemicals like that can have adverse effects on human digestive health. It is crucial for individuals to be aware of these factors and consider their own tolerance when incorporating such plants and food into their diet, as these chemicals can trigger autoimmune responses and disrupt nutrient absorption, impacting overall gastrointestinal well-being.

Psoriasis, a skin disease, causes an itchy, scaly rash, typically appearing on areas like the knees, elbows, trunk, and scalp. This chronic condition lacks a permanent remedy and causes discomfort, disrupts sleep, and lowers your concentration. Psoriasis tends to follow a recurring pattern, with periods of intensification lasting a few weeks, followed by periods of relief. Common instigators in individuals with a genetic inclination toward psoriasis encompass infections, injuries like cuts or burns, and specific medications.

My struggle with psoriasis persisted over a long period, and I must admit that, at the outset, I had deep concerns that it might be a more serious skin condition, perhaps even a form of skin cancer. The simple act of taking a shower became a painful and uncomfortable as my skin became increasingly itchy, inflamed, and characterized by prominent red patches.

The impact on my self-confidence was profound. I found myself going to great lengths to hide the visible signs of psoriasis, even resorting to growing my hair out like Tarzan to keep the affected area out of sight. It was a desperate attempt to shield myself from the judgment and scrutiny of others, as well as to regain some semblance of self-assurance.

I then thought it was a good idea to consult a medical professional about my condition. The doctor prescribed a topical steroid ointment, which I applied diligently for an entire month. I thought that this treatment would provide some relief, alleviate the symptoms, and bring back a sense of normalcy to my life. I saw little to no improvement. In fact, to my dismay, it seemed that the psoriasis was getting worse rather than better during that time. I am now free from psoriasis, and it is far easier than you'd think.

1. Calm down and relax. Find a method that calms you down, personally I go for early morning walks in nature and train hard.
2. Alcohol triggers certain immune cells called lymphocytes and skin cells called keratinocytes, as well as making the body produce substances that can cause inflammation.
3. Avoid a high inflammatory diet, I personally used the animal-based diet. I also reduced my exposure to furanocoumarins to reduce photosensitivity/photo-damage.
4. The more you puff, the more you flare. Not only is there research evidence, but whenever I smoke, I know that the next day I am going to be itchy, sore, and red.

Celiac disease is a serious autoimmune condition that develops in individuals with a genetic predisposition. When these individuals consume gluten, it causes harm to their small intestine. Over a period, this response harms the lining of your small intestine and hinders its ability to take in nutrients.

Medical researchers over time have indicated a rising trend in these occurrence rates, with an annual average increase of 7.5% observed over the past few decades. It's important to note that the examination of celiac disease incidence focuses solely on diagnosed patients, we still must take into consideration of the individuals undiagnosed.

While there isn't a known cure for celiac disease, if we apply some logic, we will know that, adhering to a strict gluten-free diet could typically aid in symptom management and promote the healing of the intestines for most individuals.

What is it about this protein that sets off a cascade of symptoms in those with celiac and even without the disease? And perhaps even more perplexing, where is this hidden gluten lurking, silently infiltrating our diets and wreaking havoc on our health? Is it in unsuspecting foods, masquerading behind labels that claim to be gluten-free? Whilst moving through this metabolic maze—why does something as common as gluten cause problems for some people? So, where is gluten hiding, sneaking into our diets even when we think we're avoiding it? Rest assured; I've got the answers you're looking for.

For individuals with celiac disease, even small amounts of gluten can trigger strong and adverse reactions. This leads to vigilant label search while shopping for packaged foods and thorough questions directed at restaurant staff to find out. Yet, it may come as a revelation that a range of products, extending beyond the realm of food, can harbour contain gluten in diverse forms.

When it comes to steering clear of gluten in **personal care products**, it's essential to be mindful of certain ingredients. Gluten can be traced back to wheat, barley, rye, triticale, and their derivatives. To make this task easier, here are some pointers:

Stay clear of ingredients with names that include wheat, gluten, or triticum (the Latin term for wheat). These encompass components like AMP-isostearoyl hydrolysed wheat protein, hydrolysed wheat protein (HWP), hydrolysed wheat gluten, triticum lipids, triticum vulgare, wheat bran extract, and wheat germ extract.

Be cautious of ingredients with barley, malt, or hordeum vulgare (the Latin term for barley) in their names, such as barley extract and hordeum vulgare extract. Keep an eye out for ingredients linked to rye or secalin cereal (the Latin term for rye).

Be aware that ingredients derived from oats or avena sativa (the Latin term for oats) may potentially be cross-contaminated with gluten. Examples include sodium lauroyl oat amino acid extract. You might not expect wheat to be involved in the production of soy sauce, but it plays a significant role in the manufacturing process. This can pose a challenge for individuals with celiac disease or gluten sensitivity. Consider switching to gluten-free soy sauce or tamari.

There's some ambiguity surrounding blue-veined cheeses. While they may employ bread mold in their production, any potential gluten content within them is exceedingly minima. However, if you're a cheese enthusiast and have issues with bleu cheese, try selecting hard cheeses as a safer alternative.

Honey isn't all the same, and in some cases, it may not even be genuine. Surprisingly, a significant portion of honey on the market is adulterated, indicating that it has been mixed with other substances such as corn syrup, glucose, or beet syrup. In certain instances, brands may even incorporate altered sugars to mimic the appearance of honey when, it is not pure honey. This is because it is cheaper to make and distribute. Rather find a local beekeeper near your home!

Like prescription medications and cosmetic products, gluten can find its way into vitamin supplements, often used as a binding agent. This means that gluten may be included in these supplements to help hold the ingredients together. It's essential for individuals with celiac disease or gluten sensitivity to carefully examine the ingredients in their vitamin supplements to ensure they align with their dietary restrictions. Additionally, consulting with a healthcare professional or pharmacist can provide valuable guidance on choosing gluten-free supplement provider.

Lupus is a serious autoimmune condition characterised by widespread inflammation within the body. The immune system, instead of safeguarding the body, mistakenly attacks and damages various tissues and organs. The symptoms of lupus can manifest throughout the body, depending on which tissues are affected. This may include the skin, blood, joints, kidneys, brain, heart, and lungs. As a result, individuals with lupus can experience a range of symptoms and complications that vary in severity and scope, making it a complex and challenging condition to manage.

Lupus is changing over time. In the UK, there are more people with lupus each year, with about 3.1% more cases annually. On the flip side, the number of new cases of lupus each year has gone down a bit, by about 1.8%, from 1999 to 2012. Also, how we decide if someone has lupus can make a difference. If we use one set of rules called the SLICC criteria, we might find more cases. But if we use another set called the ACR criteria, we might find fewer cases. So, the numbers can change depending on the rules we use to diagnose lupus. Meaning the evidence of the increase in lupus is highly inaccurate. It is still obvious there is big increase.

Why does lupus seem to affect some groups of people more than others, and could dietary factors that influence white blood cell counts be at play? It's intriguing to note that women are more likely to develop lupus, but what role might specific dietary choices have in this gender difference? Additionally, why does lupus tend to strike between the ages of 15 and 44, with only a small percentage experiencing symptoms before the age of 18? The impact of race and ethnicity on lupus prevalence raises questions as well. What dietary factors within these groups might contribute to a higher incidence of lupus, especially those influencing inflammation?

Reducing the chances of lupus flares involves making mindful dietary choices and personalizing your approach to manage this complex autoimmune condition. It's advisable to steer clear of foods containing high amounts of L-canavanine, a compound that can stimulate the immune system, potentially leading to lupus flares.

Likewise, garlic should be consumed cautiously, as it contains immune-stimulating compounds that may provoke an unwanted immune response in individuals with an already hyperactive immune system, a common characteristic of lupus.

Nightshade vegetables like eggplant, potatoes, and tomatoes are considered potential triggers for some individuals, though it's essential to recognize that lupus varies greatly from person to person.

To identify your triggers, consider going on an elimination diet under the guidance of a dietitian working with lupus patients, enabling you to point out foods that might worsen your lupus symptoms while maintaining a balanced and personalized approach to managing the condition.

As lupus can damage your skin upon exposure to UV light, we can apply similar logic to psoriasis by avoiding exposure to furocoumarins.

In conclusion, managing lupus and minimizing the occurrence of flares requires a personalized approach to dietary choices. Understanding your body's unique responses to certain foods and their potential impact on your condition is crucial. While some foods like the ones listed above have been associated with immune system stimulation, their effects can vary among individuals.

Lipedema can impact as many as 11% of women and it occurs when fat accumulates unevenly beneath the skin, typically in the buttocks and legs. While it initially presents as a cosmetic issue, it can later lead to discomfort and various complications. Lipedema is often confused with typical obesity or lymphedema.

As the lipedema advances, fat accumulation in the lower body increases, and there is potential for lipedemic fat to also accumulate in the arms.

As time passes, these fat cells obstruct the lymphatic system's vessels, which typically maintain the body's fluid balance and immune protection. This obstruction hampers the effective drainage of lymphatic fluid, resulting in the accumulation of fluid known as lymphedema.

Without appropriate intervention, lymphedema can give rise to complications like infections, slowed wound healing, the formation of fibrous tissue like scars, and the hardening of skin in the legs.

While the precise cause remains elusive, medical professionals speculate that female hormones may be a contributing factor. This hypothesis is rooted in the fact that lipedema predominantly afflicts women and frequently commences or exacerbates during puberty, pregnancy, following gynaecologic procedures, and around the onset of menopause.

Living alongside someone who has lipedema and training women with the condition has provided me with unique insights into the challenges posed by this condition. It's become clear that managing and mitigating its effects depend on adopting significant changes in diet and lifestyle. Witnessing the journey and struggle, I've come to appreciate the dedication and resilience required to make these adjustments.

Lipedema is not just a physical burden but a condition that can impact one's overall well-being. Through dietary modifications and lifestyle choices, I have seen remarkable strength and determination in a pursuit of a healthier and more comfortable life.

Their experience has underscored the importance of empathy and support in the face of such challenges, and it has instilled in me a profound respect.

When it comes down to dieting with lipedema, from my experience I saw huge differences in clients and family who stuck to a ketogenic diet or a carnivore diet. There is more evident research into why ketogenic diets are beneficial to lipedema patients, whereas there aren't as many studies as possible on carnivore.

For those struggling with lipedema, have you ever wondered how you can shed those extra pounds, boost your energy levels, and enhance your overall well-being? It's time to ask yourself: Are you prepared to take the steps necessary to achieve your weight loss goals? So, let's delve into the effective strategies, dietary choices, and training advice that can pave the way to a successful weight loss journey.

Ketogenic diets have a long history of effectively promoting rapid fat loss. They achieve this primarily by reducing insulin levels and increasing feelings of satiety through high fat intake. This dietary shift from relying on carbohydrates to using fatty acids and ketones as a source of energy sets up a favourable environment for sustainable fat breakdown, without the risk of muscle loss seen in calorie-restricted diets.

This diet can lead to reductions in adipocyte size, plasma insulin levels, and leptin levels, all of which are relevant and important to lipedema treatment. Lower insulin levels help prevent lipogenesis and adipocyte enlargement, promoting a reduction in overall adiposity.

Now the metabolic changes induced by ketosis have the potential to address the increase of adipocytes and the hyper-inflammatory response seen by reducing adiposity, lowering insulin levels to enable LI adipocyte lipolysis while suppressing appetite, and preventing the disease from overall progression.

Ketosis also showed to normalise insulin and glucose levels as well as reversing glucagon resistance. This reversal could be beneficial for lipedema patients in addressing excessive their adiposity and weight loss challenges without surgery.

Excess weight had not only affected physical well-being but had also taken a massive toll on their confidence and overall quality of life. From a trainer's perspective, I was eager to offer my support and expertise in guiding these individuals toward their weight loss aspirations. Together, we embarked on a journey of pain-free training, recognizing that sustainable progress required a holistic approach that prioritized both physical and mental well-being.

I decided to embark on a journey of learning pain-free training, specifically tailored for lipedema, through specialists in the field.

Given that lipedema can cause discomfort, pain, and limited mobility, selecting the right exercise regimen is crucial. One of the lowest-impact yet highly effective exercise options for individuals with lipedema is swimming-based activity.

Many individuals with lipedema may experience joint issues or have fragile lymphatic systems, rendering high-impact exercises like running or jumping unsuitable. Swimming-based activities are gentler on the joints, minimizing stress and enabling individuals with lipedema to engage in cardiovascular exercise without risking injury or experiencing pain.

Furthermore, swimming-based activities promote better circulation by utilizing the water's pressure to assist in moving lymphatic fluid and blood throughout the body. This enhanced circulation can help reduce swelling and alleviate discomfort in the affected areas.

As a trainer, it is essential to offer thoughtful guidance when helping individuals choose the right activity for their fitness journey. Tailoring exercise recommendations to align with an individual's specific needs, preferences, and physical condition is difficult and broad. Encouraging low-impact options, such as swimming-based activities for those with conditions like lipedema, demonstrates a commitment to their long-term health and comfort. It's about fostering a sense of empowerment, where individuals feel confident in their chosen activities and can achieve their fitness goals without risking injury or feel pain.

Cardiovascular disease causes 1 in 4 deaths in England and leads the world in causes of death and health problems. The total percentage increase in prevalent cases of total cardiovascular disease from 1990 to 2019 is approximately 93.4%. Similarly, the total percentage increase in the number of CVD deaths during the same period is approximately 53.7%.

The cardiovascular disease market is a lucrative industry, with an estimated worth of around 135 billion dollars. However, within this expansive industry, there lies a disconcerting truth: the elusive nature of the disease and its treatments often fuels speculation that the complete truth may never be fully disclosed.

There is widespread speculation that the complete truth about cholesterol's role in CVD may never be fully disclosed. The intricate interplay between cholesterol levels, dietary factors, and genetic predispositions adds layers of complexity to understanding its impact on cardiovascular health. Is it that factors beyond red meat and butter consumption are influencing the rise in cholesterol levels, contributing to clogged arteries? And amidst the cholesterol concerns, why is the often-overlooked role of triglycerides in heart health still shrouded in relative obscurity, with so few taking notice? Nevertheless, this uncertainty serves as a call to action.

There is a certain criterion which could put you at risk of potential risk and that includes having high blood pressure, elevated blood sugar levels, excess weight in the abdomen, low levels of HDL cholesterol and high triglycerides.

In a world where dietary choices are constantly scrutinized, could we have been misled about the real causes behind cardiovascular disease? While red meat has borne the brunt of blame for years, emerging research points to industrial seed oils as potential silent villains in this health crisis. Could it be that these oils, often touted as healthier alternatives, are, in fact, contributing to the very problem today?

Oxidized fatty acids derived from industrial seed oils have recently garnered attention for their potential involvement in the development of cardiovascular disease. Researcher James DiNicolantonio has introduced the "oxidized linoleic acid theory of coronary heart disease," linking the consumption of linoleic acid-rich industrial seed oils to cardiovascular disease risk. According to this theory, dietary linoleic acid from these oils becomes integrated into blood lipoproteins. The inherent instability of linoleic acid increases the likelihood of lipoproteins undergoing oxidation. Oxidized lipoproteins lose their recognition by the body's respective receptors, leading to their activation of macrophages. This activation initiates foam cell formation, ultimately contributing to the development of atherosclerosis and cardiovascular disease.

Additionally, industrial seed oils worsen cardiovascular disease risk by creating an imbalance between omega-6 and omega-3 fatty acids. A high omega-6-to-omega-3 ratio is a well-established risk factor for cardiovascular disease, as excess omega-6 promotes pro-inflammatory and prothrombotic effects within the vascular system.

Furthermore, there's a burgeoning theory suggesting that canola and soybean oils may contribute to cardiovascular disease by inhibiting processes reliant on vitamin K2, a component for heart health.

It's also important to understand how added sugars can contribute to the development of heart disease. When we consume excess added sugars, such as those found in sugary drinks, sweets, and processed foods, our bodies can face several adverse effects.

These sugars lead to an increase in blood glucose levels, causing the pancreas to release insulin to manage the excess sugar. Over time, this continuous cycle of high sugar intake and insulin production can result in insulin resistance, where the body's cells become less responsive to insulin's signals. This insulin resistance is associated with various risk factors for heart disease, including higher blood pressure, increased inflammation, and unfavourable changes in blood lipid levels.

Additionally, excessive sugar consumption can lead to weight gain and obesity, which are known contributors to heart disease. Therefore, reducing added sugar intake is a crucial step in promoting heart health.

Added sugars are metabolized rapidly by the body, often leading to what's commonly referred to as a 'sugar crash.' This occurs due to a significant surge in insulin levels, followed by a subsequent decrease in blood glucose levels. However, elements like dietary fiber, the sugars present in fruits enter the bloodstream and undergo metabolism at a considerably slower pace. These sugars demand more substantial effort from our bodies for breakdown compared to added sugars.

Cancer in its broad and daunting spectrum, represents a complex and relentless group of diseases characterized by the uncontrolled growth and spread of abnormal cells in the body. This condition can live in numerous forms, each with its own unique traits and challenges. At its core, cancer disrupts the finely tuned mechanisms that regulate cell division, leading these rogue cells to multiply uncontrollably, forming tumours or infiltrating healthy tissues and organs. The consequences are often dire, as cancer can impair the normal functioning of vital bodily systems, leading to a cascade of debilitating symptoms and, if left unchecked, potential death. The causes of cancer are multifactorial, encompassing genetic predispositions, environmental exposures, lifestyle choices, and other intricate factors.

Despite their remarkable advancements in research and treatment, cancer remains a formidable adversary, demanding ongoing efforts in prevention, early detection, and innovative therapies to confront its pervasive impact on individuals and communities worldwide.

My question is whether a cure for cancer exists but remains concealed, hidden in secrecy due to the staggering financial stakes tied to the cancer market, which is valued at approximately 205 billion dollars? The tantalising prospect of a universal cancer cure raises intriguing questions about the motives of the pharmaceutical industry, research institutions, and healthcare establishments. Could such a hidden truth fundamentally alter the course of medical history, or does it merely dwell within the realm of a so called "conspiracy theory", leaving us to ponder the truth between profit and the pursuit of a cure for one of humanity's most ruthless diseases.

I AM NOT AN EXPERT on cancer, I would like to emphasize that, in my understanding, many diseases, including cancer, often appear to be influenced by a multitude of factors. From the information I've gathered, it seems that these conditions are typically multifactorial in nature, and I tend to be sceptical of theories that propose a single, definitive cause for any given disease.

It's crucial to acknowledge the evidence that establishes cancer as a genetic disease with contributing factors. There are clear examples of inherited mutations that are undeniably linked to an elevated risk of developing cancer.

What becomes evident from this viewpoint is the connection between both inherited and non-inherited causes of cancer: problems with mitochondria. This trouble with mitochondria can be triggered by a range of cancer-causing agents, including not just genetic factors but also elements like radiation, exposure to chemicals, and dietary habits. This perspective, which bridges different causal elements, encourages us to reconsider how we perceive the complex origins of cancer.

The reason cancer becomes entangled in this metabolic maze is that it may, represent a metabolic disorder. This metabolic shift in cancer entails a departure from the usual, tightly regulated metabolic pathways, steering instead towards a less efficient yet more favourable route for the accelerated growth and proliferation of cancer cells.

Neurodegenerative disorders emerge as a complex challenge in medical science. These conditions, including Alzheimer's disease and Parkinson's disease, erode the nervous system. They cast a shadow over the lives of those affected and their loved ones. As we go through this specific metabolic maze of neurodegenerative disorders, our aim is not only to see what has happened and changed over the years to see an estimated increase of 147.95% in Alzheimer's and 100% in Parkinson's.

Considering the terrifying burden that Alzheimer's disease causes in individuals and society, there is an urgent call for proactive measures. If Alzheimer's development encompasses an infectious element, there are numerous actions you can take to reduce inflammation, commencing today, to lower your risk of developing this neurodegenerative condition.

For a long time, I questioned whether neurodegenerative disorders, have a deeper connection to our gut health, potentially involving autoimmune responses? As we have already talked about important relationship between our gut and health, we are compelled to ponder the emerging notion that conditions like Alzheimer's and Parkinson's might, in part, be influenced by inflammation or imbalances in our gut.

Gut health and its connection to immune function in relation to Parkinson's disease is gluten intolerance. There is a lot of medical literature indicating that gluten intolerance, specifically non-celiac gluten sensitivity, is noteworthy, particularly when it is associated with the presence of transglutaminase 6 (tTG6) antibodies. Transglutaminase 6 is an enzyme that exhibits significant activity in the brain. In cases where individuals with gluten intolerance also produce antibodies against transglutaminase 6, the consumption of gluten can trigger an immune response within the body. This immune response essentially leads to an attack on the transglutaminase 6 enzyme in the brain, which, in turn, contributes to neurodegenerative disease.

A growing amount of evidence is showing a connection between diabetes and Alzheimer's disease (AD), underpinned by the shared characteristics of impaired glucose regulation and altered brain function in both conditions.

Individuals with diabetes exhibit distinct cognitive deficits, including a decline in execution and processing speed, impairment in both verbal and nonverbal memory, and notable atrophy of critical brain regions which are changes that are also found in Alzheimer's disease. These c patterns not only serve as precursors of future cognitive decline but also hint at the shared neurodegenerative processes at play.

Insulin resistance exerts detrimental effects on the brain, impacting neuronal function, disrupting the balance of catecholamine neurotransmitters, and inciting neuroinflammation. These consequences potentially play a role in the progress of Alzheimer's disease, encompassing memory loss, reduced cognitive ability for judgment and communication, and alterations in personality and behaviour, including symptoms like anxiety and delusional thinking.

Male reproductive health issues are arising, there has been a 50% decline in sperm counts globally, accompanied by a worrisome deterioration in sperm quality, affecting 1 in 20 men today. This concerning issue in male fertility crisis finds its potential roots in several factors, including exposure to environmental endocrine-disrupting compounds, dietary concerns and hormonal imbalances. The overarching result is a surge in infertility cases, with one out of every six couples striving to conceive receiving a diagnosis of infertility.

The average testosterone levels in men have been experiencing a decline of approximately 1% per year. A study of this trend is evident when comparing the testosterone levels of seventy-year-old men in 1987-89 to those of even fifty-five-year-old men in 2002-04. Remarkably, the average twenty-two-year-old man today has the testosterone levels that are roughly equivalent to those of a sixty-seven-year-old man in the early 2000s! This pattern implies that your testosterone levels are considerably lower than your grandfather's. What's even more concerning is that this downward trajectory is intensifying, affecting men at much younger ages than ever before.

As we witness a decline in both testosterone levels and sperm counts, a pressing and troubling question emerges: What are causing these problems, silently eroding the male reproductive health? Is it modern lifestyles, saturated with stress, sedentary habits, and dietary choices combined with endocrine-disrupting compounds? Are environmental toxins casting an insidious shadow over our hormonal balance, and if so, to what extent? Are we moving towards a point of no return, where the ability to conceive and maintain essential male attributes hangs in the balance?

These are not just questions; they are urgent calls for investigation, for answers, and for action to stop declining testosterone and plummeting sperm counts in the name of safeguarding the future of men's health. We should all take the time to wake up to this epidemic as our future of mankind is truly at risk.

The global annual production of plastics has undergone a staggering increase, soaring from 50 million tons in the 1970s to a monumental over 300 million tons today. This exponential surge in plastic production has raised questions about its implications for our hormone health.

These endocrine disrupting chemicals expand into our bodies, affecting various aspects of our health. Research has uncovered unsettling links between EDC exposure and a spectrum of health issues, including ADHD, autoimmunity, disruptions in metabolism and in particular concern is the association between EDCs and lower sperm quality, as well as decreased testosterone levels.

Vaping is frequently marketed as a "safer" option to smoking, yet it carries its own set of risks if not more. While research on the impact of vaping on fertility is still somewhat limited, various components found in typical vape liquids, including nicotine and additives, are known to be associated with diminished sperm health.

It's essential to note that most of the existing research on vaping and male fertility has been conducted on rats, and while it does provide some compelling evidence of potential harm, there remains a large need for more studies on this dangerous e-cigarette.

A noteworthy study I read involving men revealed that 13% used e-cigarettes, (52% were cigarette smokers, 25% used snuff and 33% used marijuana.

Daily e-cigarette users, as well as daily cigarette smokers, exhibited significantly lower total sperm counts when compared to non-users. These findings underscore the potential adverse effects of vaping and smoking on male reproductive health.

Further insights from animal studies have added to our concerns. In a 2016 study, rats exposed to vape refill liquid experienced decreased testosterone levels, reduced sperm counts, and diminished sperm viability, irrespective of whether the vape liquid contained nicotine. A subsequent 2019 study on rats, this time employing nicotine-free e-cigarette liquid, suggested detrimental effects on the testes and impairment of the male reproductive system. These findings collectively emphasise the urgent need for more research to fully comprehend a long-term understanding.

The total amount evidence gathered shows a disconcerting reality: the widespread use of these nicotine-containing products is likely a significant contributor to the decreasing of reproductive capabilities in males. Hopefully this raises alarms about the rise of issues for male fertility but also opens more discussion about the potential long-term impact on future generations.

Female reproductive health issues pose a significant concern for the future, as indicated by data from the CDC. In women aged 15 to 49 who have never undergone childbirth and are in heterosexual relationships, approximately 19% encounter challenges with fertility (mostly with ovulation). This statistic evidently shows the alarming prevalence of infertility among this demographic of women.

The data reveals that women who have experienced at least one childbirth are comparatively less likely to grapple with infertility. Specifically, only about 6% of married women in the same age bracket (15 to 49 years) who have given birth face infertility issues. While this percentage is lower, it is by no means insignificant, and it emphasizes the far-reaching implications of infertility as a reproductive health concern. It is estimated that 10% to 20% of recognised pregnancies result in a miscarriage, the true figure is likely to be even higher. This discrepancy arises from the fact that a substantial number of miscarriages occur in the early stages of pregnancy, often before individuals are aware of their pregnancy.

In a woman's lifetime, approximately one out of every eight will experience a thyroid disorder. However, the problem escalates for those who have undiagnosed and untreated thyroid conditions, as they face an increased risk of developing infertility. The thyroid plays a role in regulating the levels of female reproductive hormones. When there is a imbalance in thyroid hormone levels, it can result in an irregularity in overall hormone balance.

Hypothyroidism, a condition characterised by an under-active thyroid gland, which can have a significant impact on a woman's reproductive health. This causes a hormonal imbalance, leading to various issues such as irregular menstrual cycles, heavy or prolonged bleeding, or even the absence of menstruation altogether. Moreover, hypothyroidism can result in anovulation, a condition where the ovaries do not release an egg, further complicating menstrual regularity and fertility. For women trying to conceive, this can be a distressing challenge. Furthermore, unmanaged hypothyroidism during pregnancy can affect the growth and development of the fetus, potentially impacting the health of the baby. We also can't forget that hypothyroidism during pregnancy can also heighten the risk of miscarriage or stillbirth, making it a critical issue to address for expectant mothers and their doctors.

Vaping among women can have an impact on fertility, potentially leading to reduced fertility function and causing delays in egg production and fertilization. It's important to recognize that the toxic substances found in vape liquids can be just as harmful as those present in traditional cigarettes. Studies have indicated that vaping during pregnancy may result in adverse effects on fetal development, potentially leading to growth problems in infants.

However, like men, there is currently insufficient conclusive evidence available regarding the long-term effects of vaping on female reproductive health. Nonetheless, in the short term, we are observing significant correlations on a larger scale.

As I train female clients, I always create programs based on their monthly cycles and hormone levels to ensure safe exercise. I have created a blueprint a of how to train to work with your menstrual cycle and not against it.

Phase 1: Menstruation

- Focus: Gentle Recovery
    - During your period, prioritize rest and recovery.
    - Engage in light activities like yoga, stretching, and walking.

Phase 2: Follicular Phase

- Focus: Building Strength and Endurance
    - As hormone levels rise, it's time for challenging workouts.
    - Incorporate cardio, strength training, and high-intensity workouts.

Phase 3: Ovulation

- Focus: Peak Performance
    - Hormones like oestrogen and testosterone peak during ovulation.
    - Aiming for intense workouts

Phase 4: Luteal Phase

- Focus: Mind-Body Balance
    - As hormone levels fluctuate, focus on a mix of activities.
    - Include strength training, yoga, and low-impact cardio to ensure stress management.

REVEALING INVISIBLE HEALTH RISKS

Passing on from the topic of metabolic and inflammatory diseases, we've acquired a comprehensive understanding of the intricate workings of our bodies and the factors that contribute to these conditions. Now, as we venture into this new chapter, our focus shifts towards a fascinating and often overlooked aspect of our health journey – the hidden defences concealed within the foods we consume.

Within the amount of our daily calories lie a crazy number of chemical compounds, influencing our body's defence mechanisms in profound ways. These concealed defenders possess the power to trigger inflammatory responses that may disrupt our well-being.

I want to emphasize that the intention here is NOT to stop consuming these foods entirely. Instead, the aim is to provide you with invaluable insight into what lies concealed within them. By uncovering the hidden components within our daily dietary choices, we can better comprehend how these elements have the potential to influence our body's inflammatory responses.

With this knowledge, you'll be empowered to make informed decisions about the foods you consume, allowing you to strike a balance that aligns with your health. The goal is not deprivation but rather education, enabling you to navigate your dietary choices with awareness and take proactive steps towards managing your inflammatory responses and performance for a healthier and more vibrant life.

Celery

The celery juice diet became so popular in 2018, after the book "Medical Medium Celery Juice: The Most Powerful Medicine of Our Time Healing Millions Worldwide." was released. The book advised that people should drink at least 16 ounces of celery juice for people with no chronic diseases (up to 24 ounces with a chronic disease).

The reason for people joining the celery juice trend was mainly for the anti-inflammatory effects through the plant compounds phytonutrients (apigenin, saponin, luteolin), which claim to reduce inflammation. Celery is a stem and leaf: two parts of a plant which don't want to be eaten. Celery contains certain chemicals known as furanocoumarins; a set of compounds that build up in the skin and crosslink your DNA to UV light.

The main concern here is the furanocoumarins causing photodamage. Photodamage is when your skin changes over an amount of time due to prolonged exposure to UV light.

As many good effects celery may have on your body with its anti-inflammatory effects, the hidden problems are causing inflammatory in your skin, increasing your risk of skin cancers and worsening skin conditions like psoriasis. Personally, as someone who has psoriasis, I have noticed that when I consume high quantities of celery, my skin tends to flare up.

Kale

Kale is a cruciferous vegetable from the mustard family of plants. In the 1990s kale became very popular for its nutritional value, including high amounts of vitamin A, C and K as well as minerals like calcium and iron. The big green leaves are usually used as an alternative for chips, blended into smoothies or mixed into a salad.

I could spend time discussing kale's abundant vitamin K, C, and E content, but let's not dwell on that. The truth is, kale doesn't deserve its "superfood" status, and it's important to understand why this misconception persists. So, why has kale been hyped up despite its drawbacks? Well, the kale trend really took off after Gwyneth Paltrow showcased kale chips on Ellen's show back in 2011. Since then, kale sales have soared, propelling it into the top 10 superfoods, but is it truly deserving of that title?

Kale contains chemicals we aren't told about, specifically glucosinolates combined with myrosinase when the plants are chewed. This then causes a reaction to produce isothiocynate, which is essentially a system of defence.

The problem we have here is that the process inhibits iodine consumption at the level of your thyroid in common serving sizes.

Another common plant toxin found within kale is known as sulforaphane. This compound triggers your body to make excess glutathione on its own. Now that sounds amazing due to ability to combat obesity, until you figure out that it comes with the negative effects of potentially risking your thyroxine production.

Broccoli

Broccoli, one of the most familiar and widely recognized vegetables, possesses an interesting history. Surprisingly, broccoli is not a naturally existing plant; instead, it is a product of human cultivation. Broccoli was selectively bred from its wild cabbage ancestor, with the primary objective being to make it more appealing and palatable to people.

Broccoli contains high levels of essential nutrients, such as Vitamin C. A mere cup of broccoli can supply you with 45-54% of your daily Vitamin C requirement. It's truly remarkable how such a small amount of broccoli can offer such a significant benefit. Interestingly, we often aren't informed about broccoli's goitrogenic effects, which are relatively like those of kale.

Some glucosinolates in brassica vegetables, when broken down, can produce goitrogenic compounds like goitrin and thiocyanate, which may interfere with thyroid hormone production.

Certain brassica vegetables, such as collards, Brussels sprouts, and certain types of kale, contain higher levels of goitrogenic compounds like goitrin, which could pose a greater risk to thyroid health.

However, some brassica vegetables, like turnip tops have relatively low levels of goitrogenic compounds (less than 10 μmol of goitrin per 100-g serving) and are considered to have minimal risk in terms of thyroid health.

Onion

Onions are bulbs, which are plant roots, therefore they hide away from predators trying to consume them. Have you ever wondered why onion make you cry? It's because of the sulphur containing compounds that act as a defence chemical. Historically, onions were consumed as a remedy for various conditions associated with diminished appetite, such as cancer and gastrointestinal issues.

Despite the presence of isoalliin, a crucial component in onions, our understanding of its impact on eating patterns and the brain regions responsible for regulating food consumption remains incomplete, due to the lack of scientific evidence.

Medical literature has unveiled a phenomenon: isoalliin, a compound found in onions, possesses the unique ability to stimulate a specific subset of neurons within the hypothalamic arcuate nucleus.

These neurons are particularly receptive to ghrelin, a hormone known for regulating hunger and appetite. This activation closely imitates the response seen when using ninjin 'yoeito, a traditional Japanese medicinal formulation.

This holds potential for individuals facing the issue of appetite loss. One group that stands to benefit from this finding includes those undergoing treatment with cisplatin, an anti-cancer drug known for its appetite-suppressing side effects. For these patients, the activation of ghrelin responsive NPY neurons by isoalliin offer a means to counteract the loss of appetite, potentially improving their overall status during a critical phase of their treatment.

Turmeric

Turmeric is a root which is loaded with oxalates and curcumin which have a hidden a surprisingly dark side since turmeric is used for its anti-inflammatory purposes. For many years turmeric has been used as a traditional Asian medicine.

In the last decade many studies have been published about the good effects of curcumin (the yellow-orange pigment). So therefore, it has now been sold as a dietary supplement. Studies now are starting to twist as the evidence is now showing its truths behind its beneficial effects.

When you eat curcumin, your body processes it a lot before it gets into your bloodstream. So, even if you take a lot of curcumin in pill form, your blood and tissues don't end up with high levels of it.

What we have understood from the evidence, is that you can't use curcumin effectively as a treatment, especially when taken by mouth. This is why curcumin hasn't shown strong results in treating chronic diseases.

Curcumin increases Reactive Oxygen Species, which are harmful molecules that can contribute to cancer development. While it has antioxidant effects at low concentrations, it can be harmful at higher concentrations.

It's generally recognised that curcumin does not cause significant short-term toxicity at doses up to 8 grams per day. For long-term use, a lower dose of around 0.15 grams per day.

Garlic

Like the onion, garlic is also a bulb. Garlic is also known as an allium, which produces amounts of allicin and mustard oil. These can cause significant reactions in many people.

Garlic contains a compound called allicin, which can be toxic when taken excessively. Allicin is known for its antibiotic properties and can kill both harmful and beneficial bacteria in the body. Excessive garlic use might disrupt the balance of normal body flora, potentially leading to potentially fatal infections.

Garlic, while known for its flavour and potential health benefits, it contains a complex array of sulphur compounds, numbering over 30 in total. These compounds can interact in ways within the body, leading to several notable effects, some of which can be less favourable. One significant consequence is the potential for damage to the delicate balance of your gut microbiome.

The sulphur compounds in garlic, when processed by your body, can cause changes in the composition and activity of the microorganisms in your digestive system. This can have far-reaching implications for your overall gut health and, in turn, impact your overall well-being.

Furthermore, garlic contains fructans, which can exacerbate digestive discomfort, particularly for those who are sensitive to such fermentable carbohydrates.

If you choose to incorporate garlic into your diet, it's advisable not to do so on an empty stomach.

Beetroot

Everyone has been told that beetroots are good for the blood flow. Yes, it is true as nitrates do help with vasodilation, but these beneficial compounds can be accessed without the added toxicity.

Beets are known to contain excessive amounts of lectins and phytic acid. These molecules bind with phosphorus and other positive ions like magnesium, zinc and calcium to limit vitamin absorption. Not only that, but they also contain loads of oxalates, the compound to mainly be involved in the creation of kidney stones.

Beets are naturally rich in a variety of nutrients and antioxidants, making them a valuable addition to a balanced diet. However, it's important to be aware that they also contain excessive amounts of lectins and phytic acid.

These compounds are known to bind with essential minerals like phosphorus, as well as other positively charged ions such as magnesium, zinc, and calcium. This binding action can limit the absorption of these vital nutrients in the digestive tract, leading to nutrient deficiencies if beets are consumed in large quantities over an extended period in certain individuals.

Furthermore, beets are notorious for their high oxalate content. Oxalates are compounds known to be involved in the formation of kidney stones, a condition that can have a range of unpleasant symptoms. The excessive consumption of oxalates from foods like beets can increase the risk of kidney stone development.

Nuts

Nuts are technically seeds, which would classify them as plants babies. Which would mean they have all sorts of defence chemicals in them to stop you from eating them. These include phytic acid, oxalates and ATIs.

Nuts are abundant in essential nutrients, and a growing body of research suggests that their consumption lowers the occurrence of cardiovascular disease (CVD). However, it's worth noting that nuts could potentially be a significant contributor to aflatoxin B1, a potent liver carcinogen, and the overall risk-to-benefit ratio remains uncertain.

Nuts are known for their nutritional richness. They are packed with essential nutrients like healthy fats, protein, fiber, vitamins, and minerals. Additionally, nuts are associated with numerous health benefits, including improved heart health, weight management, and reduced risk of chronic diseases like diabetes. Their positive impact on cholesterol levels and satiety further underscores their value in a balanced diet.

It's worth noting that, in most cases, the total advantages of including nuts in your diet significantly outweigh the potential negative effects associated with aflatoxin exposure. The health benefits they offer, when consumed in moderation, are well-established and can contribute to an overall improvement in your well-being.

When it comes to store-bought peanut butter, a specific concern arises. Some commercial peanut butter products may favour moldy peanuts, which can contain higher levels of aflatoxin. When these moldy peanuts are processed into peanut butter and sealed in a jar, there is a risk of aflatoxin contamination increasing over time.

Soy/Tofu

There are many defence mechanisms within seeds. In soy there are high levels of phytic acid, which is not denatured in the cooking process. This can chelate minerals in your gut preventing your absorption potential.

Soy is full of phytoestrogens, these phytoestrogens mimic oestrogen at a weaker level. They bind to your oestrogen receptors to either cause weak estrogenic activity or anti-estrogenic activity.

Available studies have found either no impact or revealed only minor detrimental effects on reproductive health. This is particularly the case for the few.

When exploring plant-based alternatives to animal products for increasing your protein intake, soybeans are often considered a popular choice. However, it's essential to understand that while soy does provide a source of protein, there are factors to consider when comparing it to animal-based proteins like meat.

One of the key considerations is the bioavailability of protein. Bioavailability refers to the extent and rate at which the body can absorb and utilize the protein from a particular source. It's true that the protein in soybeans is generally considered to be less bioavailable than that in meat. This means that when you consume soy protein, your body may not absorb and utilize it as efficiently as animal-based protein.

Soybeans come in various forms, including edamame, tofu, and natto. Each of these soy products has its unique nutritional profile and uses for different cooking techniques.

Flaxseed

Flaxseed oil and flaxseeds have witnessed a surge in popularity over the past couple of decades due to their rich omega-3 fatty acid content. Indeed, they boast the highest omega-3 levels per ounce among commonly consumed plant-based sources.

However, it's crucial to recognize that the type of omega-3 found in flaxseeds and flaxseed oil is distinct. This type is referred to as alpha-linolenic acid (ALA), which, unlike other omega-3 fatty acids like DHA, EPA, and DPA, does not directly provide these specific forms of omega-3. While ALA is indeed an essential fatty acid, particularly for those following plant-based diets, it's important to understand that the conversion rate of ALA into EPA and DHA within the human body is limited when relying solely on plant-based sources.

Typically, only a modest 1-10% of ALA is converted into EPA and DHA. As a result, individuals who exclude fish or other direct sources of EPA and DHA from their diets may find it challenging to attain optimal levels of these crucial omega-3 fatty acids, which are associated with various health benefits, including heart and brain health.

Therefore, while flaxseed oil and flaxseeds can contribute to your overall omega-3 intake, they may not provide sufficient EPA and DHA for those with specific dietary preferences or health goals.

To address this potential gap, individuals following plant-based diets or those with limited access to seafood or egg yolks, may consider alternative sources of EPA and DHA, such as supplementation.

Quinoa

Quinoa stands out for its high protein and fiber content, surpassing most conventional grains and seeds in this regard. This makes it an excellent choice for individuals seeking to increase their dietary protein intake and boost their fiber consumption, which can promote feelings of fullness and support digestive health.

It can promote feelings of fullness and support digestive health. However, there is a lesser-known aspect of quinoa which are saponins. Saponins are naturally occurring compounds found in quinoa and some other plant foods. While they are generally considered safe to consume, they can have a bitter taste and may cause digestive discomfort for some individuals. Saponins can be easily removed by rinsing quinoa thoroughly before cooking, a step often recommended to enhance its flavour and reduce any potential bitterness.

Quinoa saponins exhibit a wide range of biological activities, including molluscicidal, antifungal, anti-inflammatory, haemolytic, and cytotoxic properties. Despite these benefits, the negative aspects tend to outweigh the positive ones.

Saponins have the potential to cause irritation and inflammation in the gastrointestinal tract, resulting in abdominal discomfort. In severe cases, they can even contribute to the development of a condition known as "leaky gut."

Consuming substantial quantities of saponins can lead to more serious toxic effects, including damage to organs and systemic toxicity. The threshold for considering quinoa consumption toxic is typically observed to be more than 10.0 grams per kilogram of body weight.

Coffee

Coffee is essentially brewed from the seeds of a plant and can be thought of as "burned coffee seed water." In the case of coffee, its most prominent chemical component is caffeine. Contrary to being classified as a vitamin, caffeine is a methylxanthine compound.

While it is beloved by many, it's worth noting that caffeine consumption can lead to fluctuations in blood sugar levels. Regarding the purported "advantages" often associated with coffee, it's important to mention that neither observational epidemiology nor interventional studies provide conclusive evidence of unique benefits that cannot be achieved through other means. Practices like fasting, utilizing saunas.

Most of the coffee contains pesticides, acrylamide (a potential substance linked to cancer and neurotoxicity), mycotoxins (toxins produced by molds), and substances that inhibit opioid receptors, typically responsible for controlling pain, reward, and addictive behaviours.

Caffeine can cause an increase in cortisol secretion, particularly in individuals consuming moderate doses. Elevated cortisol levels can have implications for long-term health, potentially affecting the immune system.

If you are thriving and healthy, carry-on consuming coffee daily. From my view, SO MANY of my personal training clients cut out coffee and reported positive effects on their mental health and physical well-being.

Chocolate

One of the most beloved foods in Western society is chocolate. But have you ever wondered what chocolate really is? It's essentially prepared from burned cacao fruit seeds. Despite its origin, there's no denying that chocolate continues to captivate.

our taste buds with its exquisite flavour. Many doctors encourage eating dark chocolate as it high in antioxidants and loaded with polyphenols. These same doctors won't tell you that you the high oxalates in chocolate, the lectins and that chocolate contains theobromine. Food intolerances and allergies are linked to chronic digestive and autoimmune conditions.

One contributor to these issues may be the presence of plant lectins in various foods, including grains and legumes. Research has indicated that plant lectins can serve as external triggers, activating the NLRP3 inflammasome. This suggests that the NLRP3 inflammasome could play a significant role in inflammation-related disorders.

Chocolate consumption can pose a higher risk of increasing urinary oxalate excretion, especially in individuals with a high rate of oxalate absorption, whether they have overt intestinal disease or not. This elevated excretion can ultimately lead to the formation of kidney stones.

Theobromine primarily operates by blocking adenosine receptors, but it also exerts other crucial effects, such as reducing cell stress and modulating gene activity independently of adenosine receptors.

Beans

When I talk about beans, I include legumes and pulses. Beans became so popular because they contain two to three times more fiber than whole grains, and at least double the protein content of many common grains.

So, all we hear about is how beans are a great source of protein and people are becoming to replace them with animal sources through making assumptions off clear propaganda. You aren't told that red kidney beans have excessively high amounts of lectins when undercooked, specifically phytohemagglutinin.

This compound has been shown to cause food poisoning as well as causing cell agglutinating and mitogenic activities.

Mitogenic activity is essential for processes like tissue growth, wound healing, and immune responses. However, excessive or uncontrolled mitogenic activity can contribute to conditions like cancer, where cells divide uncontrollably.

Cell agglutination can have various biological implications, including in immunology and blood typing.

Immunology isn't all bad as it can be useful for identifying specific molecules or cells in the body. This information is crucial for blood transfusions and organ transplants.

However, in certain medical conditions, such as clotting disorders, the formation of blood clots through platelet agglutination can block blood vessels, potentially leading to heart attacks and strokes.

Seed oils

I hate seed oils, and you will too after I tell you how they are made. This does NOT include a high-quality olive oil, coconut oil or avocado oil. Seed oils are created by collecting seeds from crops such as corn, sunflowers, and soybeans.

These seeds are subjected to extreme heat, causing their fatty acids to undergo a detrimental "oxidation" process known as "hydrogenation." Subsequently, these oils undergo further processing with a petroleum-derived solvent and are saturated with a chemical concoction, all aimed at concealing their unpleasant appearance and odour.

Seed oils are rich in omega-6 linoleic acid, a polyunsaturated fat that has been shown to negatively affect mitochondrial membranes and promote the production of proinflammatory mediators. This condition can contribute to weight gain and exacerbate the development of metabolic and chronic illnesses.

Seed oil consumption can lead to the production of proinflammatory eicosanoids and cytokines. This results in redness and swelling in various areas of the body as part of the inflammatory response.

Why do we often choose industrial seed oils, which undergo a complex 14-step industrial process, over the simplicity of consuming butter? Butter, made by the straightforward process of whisking cream, offers a natural and wholesome option, while industrial seed oils can be laden with chemical additives.

Mushrooms

The most common mushrooms are portobello, white button and cremini are all from the same family. Mushrooms have their benefits as well as their downsides. In my opinion, the mushrooms listed above aren't as good as we think they are.

Mushrooms are essentially mold, so essentially, they produce levels of mycotoxins called arginine. This compound is known to be harmful to cause liver cancers in humans at high levels of exposure through the alteration of DNA. When eating mushrooms raw, these compounds are being ingested at higher amounts than cooked mushrooms.

Cooking mushrooms partially eliminates mycotoxins. The risk is still there but far less. I'm not writing this to tell you to stop eating mushrooms. I am warning you on the risk that eating raw mushrooms can be harmful to your over a long period of time.

Many doctors promote the use of mushrooms like lion's mane and chaga, which have shown improvements and reduces the risk of neurological diseases. To maximise that benefit it would be better to cook these mushrooms, so you don't get the added toxicity.

Raw mushrooms also contain high amount of chitin in their cell walls, when cooked they are partially eliminated. Chitin exposure can activate immune cells and create an immune network that results in inflammatory responses. Chronic inflammation can be detrimental to overall health and may contribute to various diseases.

SO, REMEMBER, if you decide to eat mushrooms, COOK THEM.

Bread

Bread contains gluten. Gluten is made up of two proteins known as gluetnins and giladins, which are also lectins. These carbohydrate binding proteins are very well known to cause leaky gut.

Gluten has been extensively investigated both in vitro and in vivo, utilizing animal and human studies It is well-documented to activate the immune system and stimulate the release of zonulin, a protein responsible for the cause of leaky gut.

Furthermore, research has revealed that gliadin, a component of gluten, can traverse the intestinal epithelium and subsequently appearing in the breast milk of lactating mothers. This occurrence raises concerns regarding the transfer of lectins from bread to infants through nursing. These observations prompt scientists and doctors to question the potential link between such exposure and the development of autoimmune development in infants.

Remarkably, this phenomenon doesn't seem to be exclusive to certain individuals; rather, it appears to manifest in all individuals, highlighting the pervasive nature of gluten's impact.

Contrary to the belief that fermentation processes like sourdough might eliminate problematic plant compounds, the evidence suggests that such compounds persist and may disrupt gut health and digestive processes. Now if you insist on still eating bread after this read, rather have sourdough. As it is the better option.

Rice

There are over 40,000 species of rice to exist on our planet. Which leaves me with the conclusion not all have been selected to study, but only a few. Most people in the world consume brown and white rice. The funny thing is we have told is that brown rice is better!

Before is say why it is funny, there is a clear lack of research focusing on human consumption of brown rice that includes a risk-benefit approach. The fact that brown rice contains more arsenic than white rice cannot be denied, and the human health risks associated with dietary arsenic exposure are well-established.

The health impacts of arsenic exposure are contingent upon several factors, including the form of arsenic (organic or inorganic), the level of exposure, and the individual's age.

Exposure to arsenic has been linked to various health conditions, including cancers, cardiovascular disease, diabetes mellitus, hypertension, and obesity.

If you are interested in maintaining your overall well-being and minimizing your toxin intake while still incorporating grains into your diet, white rice is the preferred choice due to its lower toxicity levels compared to other grains. This is attributed to the absence of the rice germ and bran in white rice.

For human dietary purposes, it's worth noting that fruits offer significantly higher nutritional value than rice. If consuming rice poses no concerns and inflammation in your body, you are certainly free to continue.

Oats

Oats have been a staple in the Scottish diet for over 5,500 years. Oats are very popular because they are good source of fibre called beta-glucan. We aren't told that oats have high amounts of phytic acid, oxalates and have loads of lectins.

Oats contain notably high levels of phytic acid, a naturally occurring compound that has been observed to have a significant impact on the absorption of essential minerals such as magnesium, calcium, and zinc. Phytic acid can form complexes with these minerals, making them less bioavailable for absorption by the body.

Moreover, excessive consumption of oats and oat-based products like oat-milk might disrupt your digestion due to their fiber content, which can sometimes lead to gastrointestinal discomfort or bloating in some individuals.

Many oat milk products on the market often mix oats with sugars and seed oils, resulting in a mixture that can be considered less than optimal for both personal health and the environment. This concoction is sometimes marketed as a healthier and more eco-friendly choice, but you are harming yourself and the plant.

To expand on this, inorganic oats are sprayed with glyphosate, a weed killer which is highly carcinogenic. If you are to eat oats, make sure you get them organic but there are many other carb sources to get fiber from on top the extra minerals and vitamins without added toxicity and carcinogenic effects.

Tomatoes

Tomatoes, like other members of the nightshade family. For most people, consuming ripe, red tomatoes in normal culinary quantities is not associated with toxicity. In fact, ripe tomatoes are a staple in diets around the world and are considered safe for most individuals.

The glycoalkaloid levels in ripe tomatoes are significantly lower than those in the less edible parts of the plant, contain naturally occurring compounds known as glycoalkaloids. These glycoalkaloids, including tomatine, are present in various parts of the tomato plant, such as the leaves and stems.

The bulk of the available evidence is predominantly anecdotal and stems from individual clinical experiences. However, it is noteworthy that a considerable number of people have shared their accounts of experiencing notable enhancements in a range of health concerns. These improvements encompass various issues, such as skin conditions, acne, fatigue, joint discomfort, and back pain.

From a chemical perspective, these plants possess variable concentrations of solanine, which is classified as a glycoalkaloid compound known to have adverse effects on both animals and humans. The riper the fruit the less concentration of solanine.

I am a huge fan of fruit, but out of all the fruits tomatoes are the most toxic. If you do not feel or notice changes when you eat them, then carry on doing so. If you do have any skin conditions like psoriasis or eczema, then cutting out tomatoes would not be a bad due to its lectin content as well. `

Eggplant

Did you not know eggplants are fruits? Funny enough they are considered as berries. Eggplants contain appreciable amounts of nutrients which gives it beneficial effects. Now eggplant is not actually popular for its nutrients, but for the taste and texture in certain cuisines. So, it's purely just to satisfy your palette. It's important to highlight the potential toxicity of certain plants within the context of their chemical composition, which includes compounds like glycosides, saponins, and protocatechuic acids.

Among these compounds, glycosides are notable for their potential to have adverse effects when consumed in excessive quantities. For instance, glycosides found in certain plants can lead to ventricular contractions, which, in extremely rare cases, can result in fatal poisoning. However, it's crucial to realise that the amount of the plant consumed would need to be exceptionally high for such severe effects to occur.

In practical terms, the likelihood of experiencing toxic effects from glycosides in everyday dietary consumption of plants like eggplant is exceedingly low. To put it in perspective, typical culinary uses of eggplant, even in larger quantities, would not introduce glycosides in amounts that could negatively impact the body.

The saponin content in eggplant is quite high, even in low doses you can expect abdominal discomfort and, in some cases, diarrhoea and nausea. I've learned this from experience as well as analysing medical literature.

Potatoes

White potatoes, as part of their natural composition, contain glycoalkaloids, specifically solanine and chaconine. These compounds are notorious for their toxic properties, posing substantial risks to not only humans but also various other species.

Potatoes are so popular because of their vitamin content containing every vitamin but A and D. This sounds amazing as they are nutrient dense, but we aren't told about their dangerous phytochemicals listed above. Solanine, a potentially hazardous compound found in potatoes, especially in sprouts and specific conditions, this justifies further examination to understand its effects on the human body.

When solanine is ingested through eating potatoes, it poses a lesser risk compared to direct injection into the body. This is mainly because the body does not absorb it efficiently, it is quickly eliminated, and it undergoes transformation into a less harmful form within the stomach.

However, it's essential to note that solanine poisoning can still result in significant health issues, including severe stomach problems, nerve-related symptoms, and skin complications.

But what about sweet potatoes? While sweet potatoes do contain some of the same toxic compounds, the levels are generally lower. As such, consuming sweet potatoes in moderation is generally considered safe. However, it's important to acknowledge that there are superior sources available that offer a wider range of nutrients while maintaining lower toxicity levels.

NON-TOXIC FOOD LIST

PROTEIN	FATS	CARBS
LAMB	OLIVES	HONEY
BEEF	YOGHURT	MAPLE SYRUP
PORK	CHEESE	BERRIES
FRESH FISH	MILK	BANANAS
EGGS	LARD	MELONS
DEER	SUET	ORANGES
ORGAN MEAT	EGG YOLK	DATES
BONE BROTH	OLIVE OIL	CUCUMBER
LOW-PUFA CHICKEN	BUTTER	MANGO
	COCONUT OIL	PAPAYA
	BONE MARROW	PINEAPPLE
	AVOCADO	SWEET POTATO (IF TOLERATED)
		PEARS
		SQUASH

READ YOUR LABELS

In a world filled with health-conscious marketing and trendy diets, it's easy to be misled by labels promising health. Superfoods, low-fat products, and sugar-free alternatives fill our shelves, but do we truly understand what lies beneath these seemingly benevolent exteriors? Are we unwittingly consuming ingredients that could be contributing to inflammation, the silent precursor to a range of health issues?

My clients have often shared with me their enthusiasm for zero-calorie foods, a temptation I too once gave into until I began reading and researching product labels. It's astonishing how something seemingly harmless can hide a plethora of artificial ingredients and sweeteners, which, while calorie-free, may have detrimental effects on our health in the long run.

As I delved into the world of studying nutrition and educated myself on the importance of whole non-toxic, unprocessed foods, I learned that making informed choices is far more valuable than simply focusing on calorie counts. Now, armed with knowledge, I guide my clients toward a more balanced and nourishing diet that prioritizes the quality of ingredients over mere numbers on the nutrition labels.

As we step into this new chapter, the focus on a compelling and often overlooked dimension of our diet lies, hidden foods residing within our pantry and fridge items, seemingly healthy but containing hidden items that may jeopardise our well-being. These hidden foods, often deemed as "healthier" choices, can subtly contribute to health concerns and disrupt our bodies.

It's quite funny how butter has often been demonised as the "bad oil" for so many years, while many people remain blissfully unaware of the presence of industrial seed oils lurking in numerous butter products. These seed oils, often high in omega-6 fatty acids, can be detrimental to our health when consumed in excess. Yet, they have found their way into butter and spreads, giving them a misleading health halo. As we continue to shed light on the importance of reading ingredient labels and opting for real, minimally processed foods, it becomes evident that the old perception of butter as the villain might need a change. It's a reminder that not everything is as it seems in the world of nutrition, and staying informed is key to making healthier dietary choices.

What butter should **NOT** look like

Ingredients: **MILK (50%), RAPESEED OIL (25%)**

What butter **should** look like:

Ingredients: Organic Butter

It's quite amusing how people have an enduring love affair with chocolate, indulging in its rich, sweetness without often realizing that many chocolate products contain industrial seed oils. While chocolate itself can offer some pleasure and even potential health benefits in moderation, the addition of these less-than-desirable oils can turn a delightful treat into a stealthy source of hidden ingredients. It's a reminder that even our favorite indulgences can come with surprises, underscoring the importance of reading labels and choosing high-quality chocolate products that prioritize the use of no hidden vegetable fats or seed oils.

What chocolate should **NOT** look like:

Ingredients: Vegetable oil, soy lecithin, glucose syrup.

What chocolate **should** look like:

Ingredients: Cocoa butter, Organic cocoa mass, organic unrefined coconut sugar, Cocoa solids 70% minimum

It's common for many to purchase pre-mixed spices, but what often goes unnoticed is the amount of unnecessary and potentially questionable ingredients that can sneak into these convenient blends. While pre-mixed spices may offer convenience, they can also contain additives, preservatives diminish the purity and authenticity of the flavors. Opting to buy individual spices and mixing them yourself not only allows for better control over the flavor profile but also ensures that you know exactly what's going into your dishes. This approach not only guarantees a fresher and more vibrant taste but also empowers you to craft your own unique seasoning combinations, tailored to your taste and dietary needs, while avoiding unwanted additives that pre-mixed spices may contain.

What to **avoid** in spices:

Ingredients: Maltodextrin, potato starch, corn flour, vegetable oil.

What spices are **friendly**:

Ingredients: Any spice that doesn't contain anything but the sole ingredients for example, cinnamon contains cinnamon only.

Many people purchase protein products in pursuit of health and muscle gains, but they often fail to realize that some of these products may harm their well-being and fitness progress. It's crucial to scrutinize the ingredients in these protein offerings, as some may be loaded with sugars, artificial additives, and unhealthy fats. A perfect example of this concern can be seen in the Grenade and Oreo co-branded protein bar below.

While the idea of indulging in a protein bar with the flavours of an iconic cookie might be deemed healthier, it's crucial to delve deeper and examine the ingredient list carefully.

Without doing so, one might inadvertently consume a product that contains more than just protein and flavour. Therefore, it's important to exercise caution and conduct thorough research before making dietary choices to ensure that what you consume aligns with your fitness goals while avoiding potential health setbacks.

What protein to **avoid:**

Ingredients: More than one ingredient including gums, sweeteners, raising agents, oils, emulsifiers and starches.

Which protein to **get:**

Ingredients: 100% organic grass-fed unflavoured whey protein

Avoid Zero Calorie

Zero-calorie foods rely on artificial sweeteners to mimic the taste of sugar without the calories. However, these sweeteners can disrupt our body's ability to regulate calorie intake, potentially leading to overconsumption of calorie-dense foods. Artificial sweeteners may interfere with metabolism, potentially causing weight gain and an increased risk of metabolic disorders like diabetes. They can also trigger cravings for sugary, high-calorie foods.

Emerging research suggests that artificial sweeteners can negatively impact our gut microbiome, which plays an essential role in digestive health and overall well-being. Alterations in gut bacteria can promote inflammation and metabolic disturbances. Consuming zero-calorie foods filled with artificial additives can.

trigger inflammation in the body, which is linked to various health issues, including heart disease and autoimmune disorders. Zero-calorie foods can show an unhealthy relationship with food, encouraging restrictive eating patterns and an obsession with calorie counting that may lead to eating disorders.

These foods often contain synthetic chemicals and additives, which may have unknown long-term health consequences and can be problematic for individuals with sensitivities or allergies. Food manufacturers often market zero-calorie products as "healthy" or "weight-friendly," but the absence of calories doesn't necessarily equate to a lack of negative health effects. Instead of relying on zero-calorie foods, prioritise whole, minimally processed, and nutrient-dense options. These foods provide essential nutrients, satisfy hunger, and reduce cravings, promoting a balanced and sustainable approach to eating.

THE FITNESS PUZZLE

My thorough research in human anatomy and biology has led me to the missing piece of the puzzle in the metabolic maze– training is the missing piece that contributes to the worlds of inflammatory responses and fitness.

The human body is an awe-inspiring and complex biological machine, made to perform a bunch of functions, including the regulation of inflammation. Inflammation, while often perceived negatively, is a fundamental component of our immune system's defence mechanism. It plays a pivotal role in safeguarding the body against pathogens and injuries. However, when inflammation becomes chronic or excessive, it can lead to a range of health issues, including cardiovascular diseases, autoimmune disorders, and metabolic disorders.

Exercise, in all its forms, exerts an influence on the body's physiological systems. Notably, it has been demonstrated that regular physical activity can modulate inflammation in various ways. Exercise prompts the release of anti-inflammatory cytokines, while also enhancing the sensitivity of cells to insulin, which plays a pivotal role in glucose regulation.

Fitness, characterised by improved cardiovascular endurance, muscular strength, and overall physical performance, is connected to an individual's metabolic health. Training, as the cornerstone of fitness, induces adaptations in the body that enhance its ability to handle inflammatory responses. The metabolic maze begins to unravel as we realize that training is the catalyst for these adaptations.

Weight training is the quickest way to achieving changes in your body. If your goal is to transform your physical appearance – a goal that often serves as a powerful motivator for many individuals – nothing will ever surpass the effectiveness of resistance training. Secondly, I'd like to underscore the significance of resistance training when executed correctly. It's highly adaptable to individual needs and preferences, whether you opt for weights, cables, machines, or even bodyweight exercises. This adaptability sets it apart from other forms of exercise, making it a standout choice. When tailored to an individual's specific requirements, resistance training has the remarkable ability to rebalance hormones.

In situations where my client presents symptoms of chronic fatigue, it's crucial to avoid an excessive focus on cardio exercises. Cardiovascular workouts can, in many instances, have counterproductive effects. For instance, if someone is experiencing low testosterone symptoms, traditional resistance training is unmatched in its capacity to boost testosterone levels. An excessive amount of cardio exercise may have the opposite effect by potentially reducing anabolic hormone production.

Resistance training plays a pivotal role in achieving hormonal equilibrium. It has the capacity to harmonize the secretion of growth hormones and testosterone, with documented impacts on oestrogen and progesterone levels in women. In the context of the Modern Western lifestyle, it stands out as an exceptionally effective method of engaging the body and achieving desired results.

Lastly, the relationship between muscle mass and the efficient circulation of lymphatic fluid within the body is a critical factor in our overall health.

Essentially, the less muscle mass one has, the slower the movement of lymphatic fluid, which is responsible for eliminating toxins and waste from our system. To promote longevity and, it's important to engage in a regular regimen of safe, heavy lifting exercises for a minimum of three days per week. These exercises not only contribute to the development of muscle mass but also facilitate the flow of lymphatic fluid, aiding in the body's detoxification process. By having a routine that prioritises muscular strength and health, we can pave the way for a longer and healthier life, ensuring our bodies are well-equipped to fend off the detrimental effects of toxins.

The reason behind this less muscle mass resulting in reduced lymphatic fluid circulation is due to the integral role muscles play in the lymphatic system's functioning. Muscles serve as pumps for the lymphatic system, facilitating the movement of lymphatic fluid through muscular contractions. When muscles contract, they compress nearby lymphatic vessels, promoting the flow of lymphatic fluid. This contraction and relaxation of muscles create a pumping action, aiding in the prevention of tissue swelling.

The profound connection between weight training and overall health serves as a metabolic currency that pays dividends throughout one's life. Weight training not only helps sculpt a stronger and more resilient physique but also fosters a robust metabolic system.

Cardiovascular training offers its own set of health benefits, no doubt about it. However, within the context of a human living a sedentary lifestyle or even without, our primary objective is to elevate metabolic rates. In our hunter-gatherer setting with scarce food resources, an accelerated metabolism might not be advantageous.

However, in in modern lifestyle, where food is available 24/7, and desk jobs are common, enhancing your metabolism becomes an asset in navigating daily life. If you live or even don't live a sedentary lifestyle engaging in regular cardiovascular exercise, such as jogging, yoga, or dancing, holds a tremendous of health benefits. Striving for just 150 minutes of moderate-intensity activity each week, where effort levels range from 50 to 70 percent of your maximum capacity, can significantly enhance your overall well-being. If you don't take part in cardio activity, then even just walking a minimum of 8000 steps per day in acceptable. These benefits encompass improved cardiovascular health, weight management, enhanced respiratory function, and mental well-being, including stress reduction and alleviation of symptoms related to anxiety and depression.

Cardio will also contribute to musculoskeletal strength and flexibility, better sleep, improved cognitive function, increased longevity, and enhanced bone health, particularly in activities like jogging. Furthermore, it often facilitates social interactions, fostering a sense of community and emotional well-being. Although cardiovascular activities can yield contrasting effects. Engaging in extensive and excessive cardio prompts the body to optimize calorie expenditure efficiency. Essentially, it signals to the body, "We're expending significant calories due too much activity; so, you need to become more efficient in calorie utilisation."

Over time, consistently engaging in excessive cardio routines can lead to a reduction in calorie burn during activity as the body becomes adept at conserving energy. Essentially, what occurs is that the body becomes proficient at not burning calories to the extent that it also results in a decrease in calories burned at rest. This can potentially lead to weight maintenance or even weight gain despite increased levels of physical activity, as the body becomes highly efficient in preserving energy, which may be detrimental for those aiming to manage or lose weight.

It becomes abundantly clear that cardio exercises should be regarded as a valuable and indispensable element of a healthy lifestyle. Their capacity to promote cardiovascular health, enhance mental well-being, and contribute to overall physical fitness is beyond dispute.

The importance of moderation and a customised approach cannot be overstated when incorporating cardio into one's routine. Every individual's fitness journey is unique, shaped by their specific goals, body type, and lifestyle. What works effectively for one person might not be suitable for another. Hence, tailoring the intensity, duration, and type of cardio exercise to suit one's individual needs becomes essential.

In the pursuit of optimal health, the principle of moderation is important. While regular cardio can provide an array of benefits, pushing the boundaries into excessiveness may inadvertently lead to unanticipated consequences. Prolonged and intense cardio can strain the body, increasing the risk of overuse injuries, fatigue, and diminishing returns in terms of calorie burn.

Mobility training is often forgot about. A decrease in mobility can have significant implications for inflammatory disorders. Myofascial tissue, a component that lines our muscles, tendons, and organs, establishes vital connections with our bones. This intricate network, intertwined throughout the body, operates as a unified system. When the fascia loses its suppleness and flexibility, it can give rise to discomfort and pain.

Our body relies on a complex network of highly adaptable fibers, intricately linked to one another. To maintain the functionality and well-being of fascia, other essential elements such as water and hyaluronic acid come into play. Elastic connective tissue, constituting around 70% water, collaborates with hyaluronic acid, which functions as a lubricating agent within our connective tissues. These molecules have the remarkable ability to interconnect and form structures resembling a sponge, adept at attracting water particles.

Consequently, when there is a decline in hyaluronic acid levels, our connective tissue loses its mobility and suppleness, potentially sets off health issues. This diminished mobility not only affects the functioning of our fascia but can also disrupt the intricate balance of inflammatory responses due to stiffness, potentially leading to the development or worsening of inflammatory disorders like arthritis. Therefore, preserving the health and flexibility of our fascia through proper hydration and the maintenance of essential molecules like hyaluronic acid becomes imperative to support overall well-being and mitigate the risk of inflammatory complications.

Using myofascial release using tools like foam rollers, a transformative process happens within the body. This process involves the reorganisation of collagen fibers within the fascia, setting in motion a cascade of beneficial effects.

When myofascial release techniques are applied, the collagen fibers within the fascia reorganise. This reorganization allows for improved flexibility and suppleness, enabling the fascia to regain its natural capacity for movement and function.

These techniques stimulate fibroblasts, specialised cells within the body, to reinitiate the production of hyaluronic acid. Hyaluronic acid plays a pivotal role as a lubricating agent within the connective tissue, and its resurgence is instrumental in restoring optimal fascial health. This production of hyaluronic acid effectively transforms the fascial network into a new reservoir of moisture, healing the tissue.

As a result of these processes, the fascia regains its ability to glide smoothly and efficiently. This newfound mobility not only promotes physical comfort and flexibility but also contributes to overall well-being. The restoration of proper fascial function aids in reducing the risk of inflammation-related disorders and supports improved lymphatic flow.

I always teach my clients this approach as it fosters a quicker recovery but also leads to a range of motion within the joints and muscles that may have been restricted or compromised.

THE ROAD TO RELIEF

I had been on a strict diet for what felt like an eternity, counting calories and restricting myself from indulging in the simple pleasures of delicious meals. While I had initially embarked on this dietary journey with the best of intentions—to get down to 8% bodyfat.

As time went on, I noticed subtle changes in my body, ones that I couldn't quite comprehend. Fatigue settled to the point where I was waking up more tired than I was going to bed. I also noticed a shift in my mood, a persistent frustration that made everything around me give me a feeling of anger. But perhaps the most concerning change of all was the unsettling silence from a part of my body that had always been quietly reliable—the sudden shutdown of my testes.

Alarmed and bewildered, I delved into research, spending countless hours scouring articles, medical journals, and forums in search of answers. It was during one of these late-night searches for knowledge that I stumbled upon the conclusion—my prolonged dieting had disrupted my hormone balance to such an extent that it had led to the complete shutdown of my testes.

After hours of research, I discovered the right ingredients that could help me regain my hormonal balance. With each passing day, I experimented with various combinations of foods crafting smoothies that could benefit the situation.

Within just 14 days of my effort, I noticed a profound change within myself. My energy levels surged, and the clouds of fatigue lifted, revealing a renewed sense of vitality. My mood brightened, and I felt more like myself than I had in a long time. Most importantly, the silent testes stirred back to life, signalling that my hormone levels were indeed balancing out.

The following pages contain 35 different toxin-free juice and smoothie recipes. You can adjust the consistency to your liking by adding water and ice, as everyone's preferences differ!

Male reproductive health & Muscle Gain Shake

Ingredients:

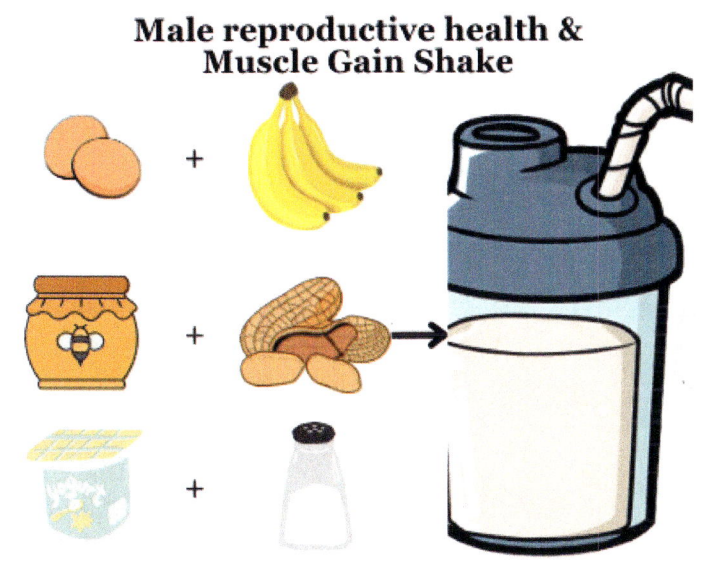

- 4 eggs
- 1 eggshell
- 2 bananas
- 1 tbsp Honey
- 1 tbsp Peanut Butter
- 2 grams salt
- 2 tbsp yogurt

This shake, which I used to address my hormone problems and promote muscle gain. This shake is beneficial for increasing blood flow, raising luteinizing hormone levels, enhancing muscle mass, and is packed with antioxidants that neutralize free radicals, which can potentially damage sperm

Female reproductive health

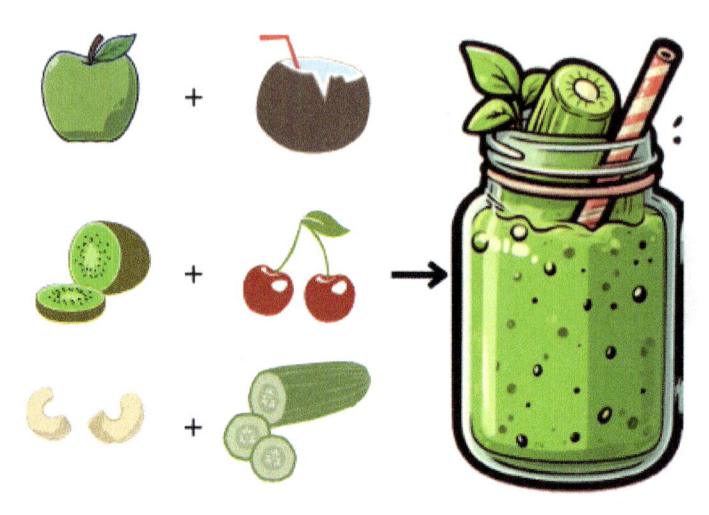

Ingredients:

- 1 apple
- 1 kiwi
- 30g cashews(optional)
- 1.5 cups coconut water
- 0.5 cups cherries
- 1/4 cucumber

Researchers at the Harvard School of Public Health highlighted the significance of omega-3 fatty acids by observing that women who incorporated the highest levels of monounsaturated fats into their diets during the IVF cycle exhibited a remarkable 3.5-fold increase in the likelihood of achieving a successful pregnancy.

Cherry lime Pre-workout

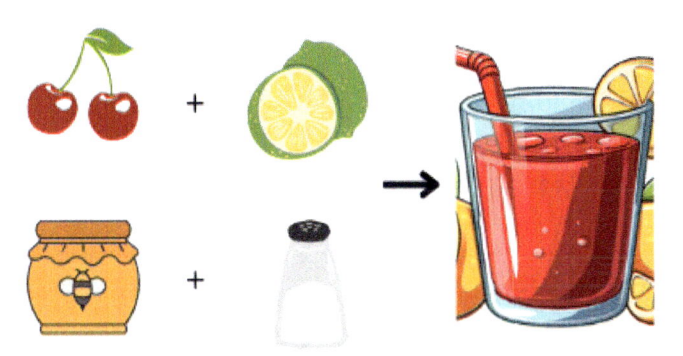

Ingredients:

- 1 tsp honey
- 1/2 lime juice
- 1/2 tsp salt
- 1/2 cup cherries

When working out, our muscles can experience exercise-induced damage due to a combination of factors, including mechanical stress and immune system responses. This immunological stress is often driven by inflammation and heightened oxidative activity. Cherries are a natural source of anthocyanin, a phenolic compound that offers potential antioxidant and anti-inflammatory properties when consumed. This dynamic trio of cherries, honey, and salt can help counteract the effects of exercise-induced muscle damage, supporting muscle contraction with increased blood flow and mitigating the impact of stressors associated with physical activity.

Waterlime Pre-workout

Ingredients:

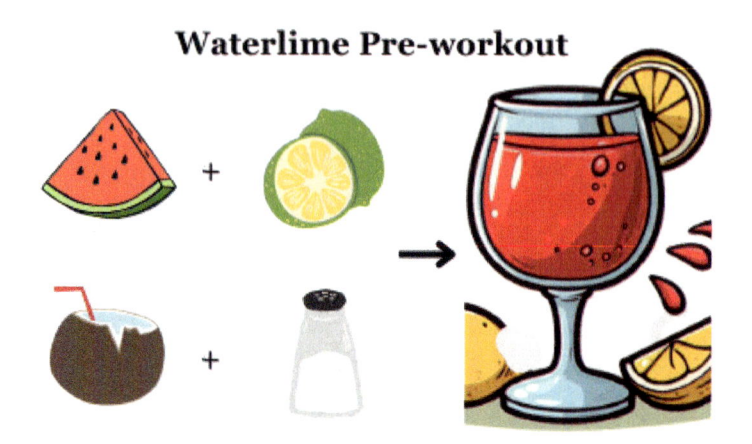

- 1 cup watermelon
- 1 cup coconut water
- 1/2 tsp salt
- 1/2 lime juice

I find that dehydration ruins training a lot of the time, so we need to make sure that we are filled with electrolytes. This watermelon juice serves as an effective electrolyte balancer, enhancing its suitability as a pre-workout drink. This leads to enhanced endurance exercise performance and a notable increase in post-exercise antioxidant levels. To maximize its advantages, consider consuming this 45 minutes before your workout to provide you the benefits.

Berry Blast Pre-workout

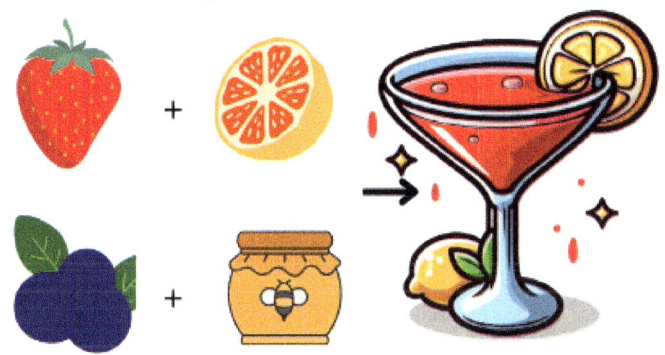

Ingredients:

- 1/2 cup strawberries
- 1 grapefruit
- 1 tsp honey
- 1/2 cup blueberries

Incorporating grapefruit into the mix for enhanced electrolyte balance, this blend harnesses the power of berries to boost performance. Berries, known for their antioxidant-rich profile and natural sugars, make them an ideal addition. Blueberries contains polyphenolic content, that can combat post-exercise muscle fatigue. So, when you're gearing up for a workout, this mixture of berries and grapefruit promises to be a valuable addition to your fitness, boosting not only your performance but also your overall well-being.

Follicle Fuel Infusion

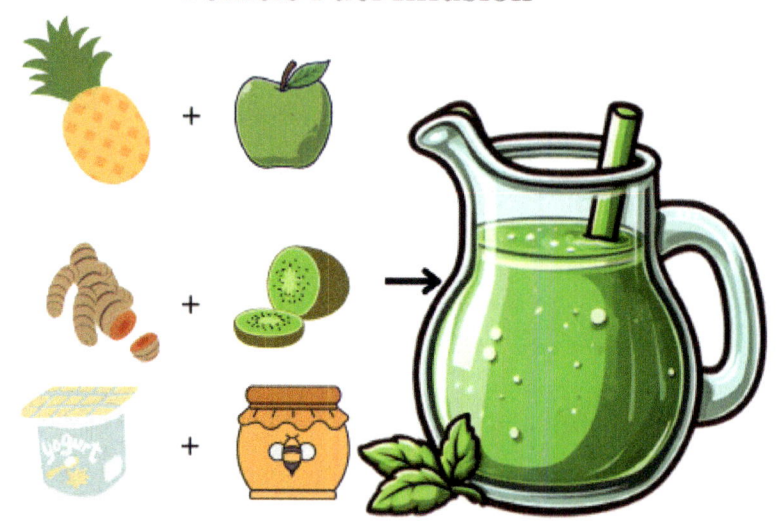

Ingredients:

- 1 kiwi
- 1/2 cup pineapple
- 1/2 tsp tumeric
- 2 tbsp yogurt
- 1 tsp honey
- 1/2 green apple

Will a smoothie cure your hair loss? Possibly not, but ensuring your getting the right nutrients you can prevent it. The yogurt in this acts as a animal based vitamin B5 source which prevents the thinning of your hair through increased blood flow. With my psoriasis, turmeric in low dosages worked amazing with its anti-inflammatory properties to reduce skin irritation. The Vitamin C content in the pineapple will prevent severe hair fall through fighting free radicals.

Citrus Psoriasis Relief

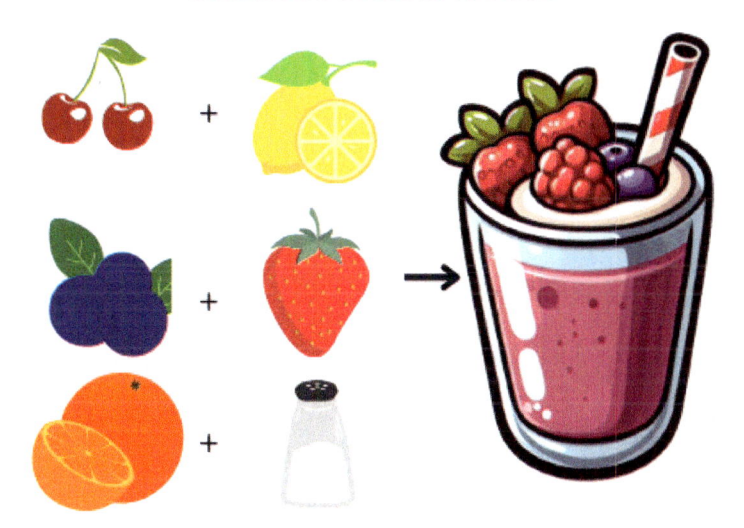

Ingredients:

- 1 cup orange juice
- 1/3 cup cherries
- 1/3 cup of strawberries
- 1/3 cup blueberries
- 1/2 squeezed lemon
- 1.5g salt

Each ingredient plays a vital role in reducing inflammation in its unique way. cherries are rich in antioxidants, which can help neutralize harmful free radicals that contribute to inflammation. The combination of strawberries and blueberries adds a burst of anti-inflammatory phytochemicals and vitamins to the mix. Lemon juice not only enhances the flavor but also provides a refreshing dose of vitamin C, known for its anti-inflammatory properties.

The common cold blend

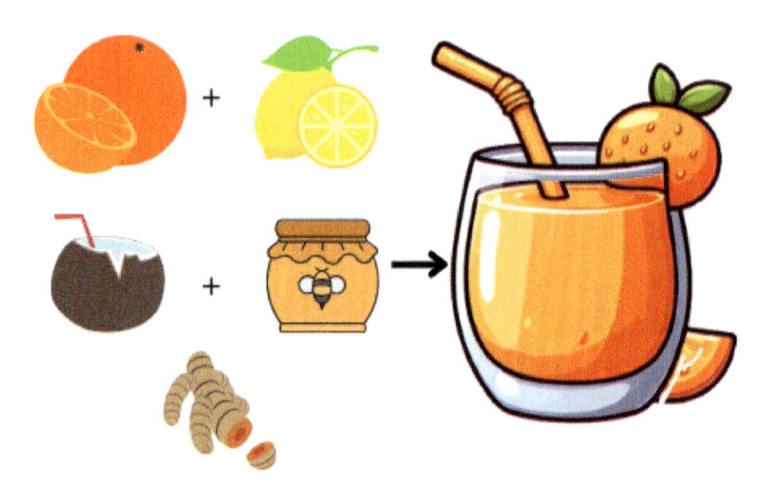

Ingredients:

- 2 oranges
- 1 lemon
- 1/2 tsp turmeric
- 1 tsp honey
- 200ml coconut water

Each ingredient plays a vital role in promoting a strong immune response. Oranges and lemons are loaded with vitamin C, which is crucial for boosting the immune system and shortening the duration of your cold. Turmeric, with its potent anti-inflammatory and antioxidant properties, can help alleviate congestion and reduce inflammation in the throat and sinuses. The element of honey provides soothing relief for a sore throat, while coconut water replenishes lost fluids and electrolytes from dehydration.

Kidney clean

Ingredients:

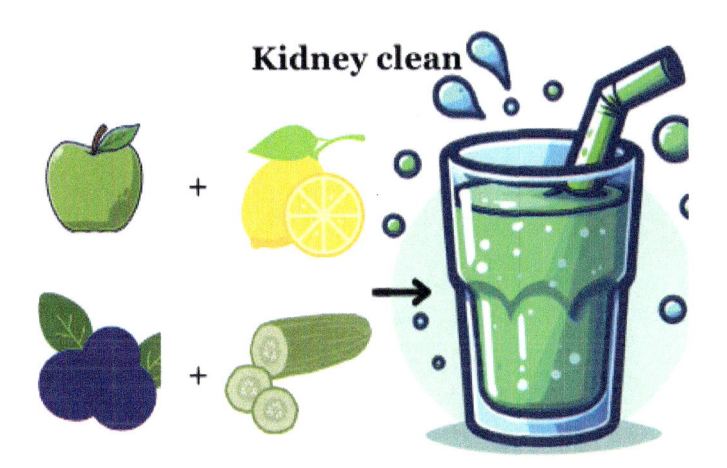

- 1 apple
- 1/4 cucumber
- 1/2 cup blueberries
- 1 lemon

The apple's fibrous content aids in opening the liver's ducts, facilitating the removal of toxins and waste materials. Cucumbers have uric acid-reducing compounds, plays a role in preventing conditions like gout by supporting the elimination of excess uric acid. Lemon, rich in vitamin C, stimulates the production of vital liver enzymes necessary for detoxification. Blueberries, abundant in antioxidants, act as guardians against oxidative stress. By countering harmful free radicals, they guard the liver from damage and uphold its optimal function.

Metabolism booster

Ingredients:

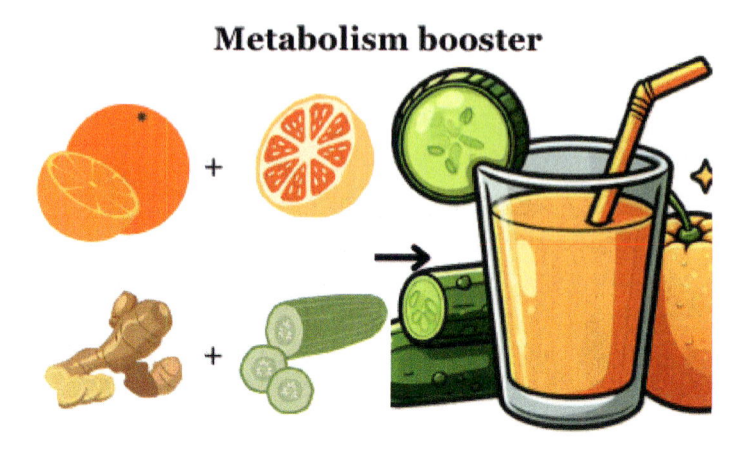

- 1 grapefruit
- 1 orange
- 2g ginger
- 1/4 cucumber

Grapefruit, rich in vitamin C and antioxidants, boosts your metabolism, making it more efficient at burning fat. The orange, also brimming with vitamin C and dietary fiber, aids digestion and contributes to healthy skin. The addition of 2g of ginger, known for its anti-inflammatory properties, not only enhances digestion and reduces bloating but also plays a role in stimulating fat-burning processes. When combined with the hydrating qualities of a cucumber, this drink metabolically activates your body.

Brain fog fix

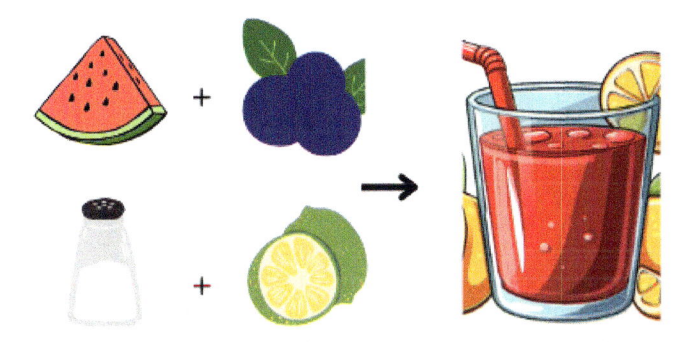

Ingredients:

- 1 cup watermelon
- 1 lemon
- 1 cup blueberries
- 1/2 tsp salt

Watermelon is a natural source of L-citrulline, an amino acid known for its role in boosting nitric oxide production. This nitric oxide, in turn, plays a pivotal role in dilating blood vessels and enhancing blood flow. Improved blood circulation to the brain facilitates superior oxygen and nutrient delivery, a vital factor in maintaining clear and sharp thinking while preventing brain fog. Moreover, the addition of electrolytes, particularly sodium in the salt, aids in regulating fluid balance within the body. Meanwhile, the blueberries, packed with flavonoids and antioxidants, reduce forgetfulness and mild confusion.

The natural laxative

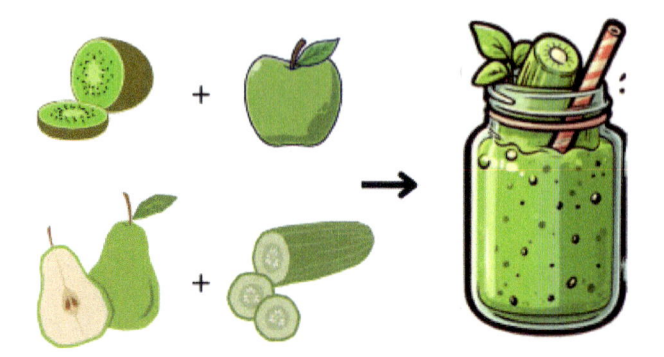

Ingredients:

- 1 pear
- 1 apple
- 1 cucumber
- 2 kiwis

If you find yourself popping your head veins on the toilet, it's a sign you need this drink. Pears, with their higher fructose content and the presence of sorbitol, a sugar alcohol, serve as a gentle natural laxative. Cucumbers, on the other hand, offer an array of health benefits, including stabilizing blood sugar levels and maintaining optimal hydration. Their abundant fiber and water content play a crucial role in promoting regularity and preventing constipation. Meanwhile, kiwis, low in calories, contribute to weight management by fostering healthy digestion. As for the apple, it provides a gentle laxative effect by easing bowel movements.

Liver clean

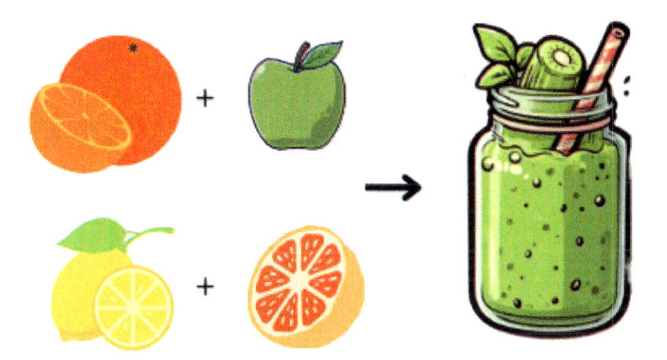

Ingredients:

- 1 orange
- 1/2 apple
- 1 lemon
- 1 grapefruit

When your kidneys are unable to effectively remove waste products from your blood, your liver steps in to assist. This situation can put extra strain on your liver, as it needs to process and detoxify substances that the kidneys would typically eliminate. Lemon juice can stimulate the production of liver enzymes that help eliminate toxins from the body. Grapefruit contains compounds that can help reduce inflammation in the liver, promoting its overall health. The fiber in oranges may also help regulate cholesterol levels in the liver. Apples contain pectin, a substance that helps cleanse the digestive system, indirectly benefiting the liver.

Stomach soother

Ingredients:

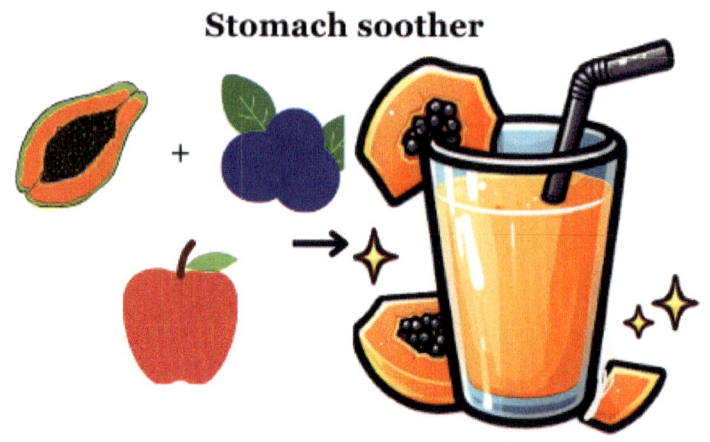

- 1/2 papaya
- 1 cup blueberries
- 1 red apple

Stomach ulcers form within the stomach lining and can arise due to factors like smoking, excessive alcohol intake, and the frequent use of anti-inflammatory drugs. This particular juice is not only good to your stomach but may also offer relief for ulcers. Papayas possess properties that can help reduce the size of stomach ulcers and may even contribute to their prevention. Blueberries are abundant in antioxidants, which play a role in reducing the risk of infections. Apples have the ability to lower stomach acidity, alleviating discomfort and bloating associated with ulcers.

Joint Health Booster

Ingredients:

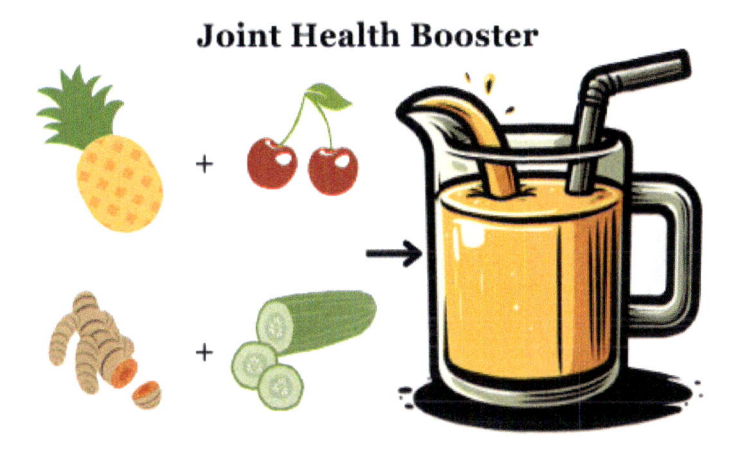

- 1/2 cup cherries
- 1/2 cup pineapple
- 1/2 cucumber
- 1/4 tsp turmeric

Cherries are rich in antioxidants, known for their inflammation-reducing properties, which can be particularly beneficial for joints. Pineapple is a source of bromelain, an enzyme recognized for its strong anti-inflammatory effects. Cucumber not only adds hydration but also offers a refreshing element to the mix. Additionally, turmeric, containing the active compound curcumin, can provide relief from joint discomfort when used in appropriate, low doses. This combination of ingredients creates a blend that supports joint health and alleviates inflammation.

Respiratory Health Blend

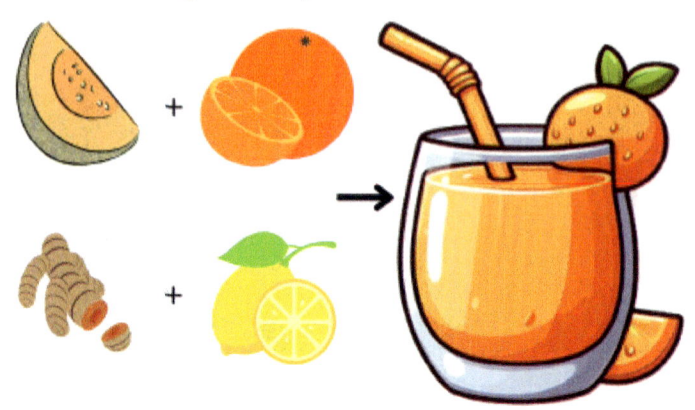

Ingredients:

- 1 orange
- 1/2 cantaloupe
- 1/2 lemon
- 2g ginger

Oranges, abundant in vitamin C, are a rich source of essential antioxidants that play a vital role in maintaining the health of your air passages. Cantaloupe, contributes much-needed hydration to this blend. The inclusion of lemon adds an extra dose of vitamin C, enhancing the overall immune-boosting benefits. However, the true standout in this blend is ginger, celebrated for its potent anti-inflammatory and decongestant properties. Ginger is a remarkable addition for providing effective respiratory relief at a low dosage.

Thyroid optimiser

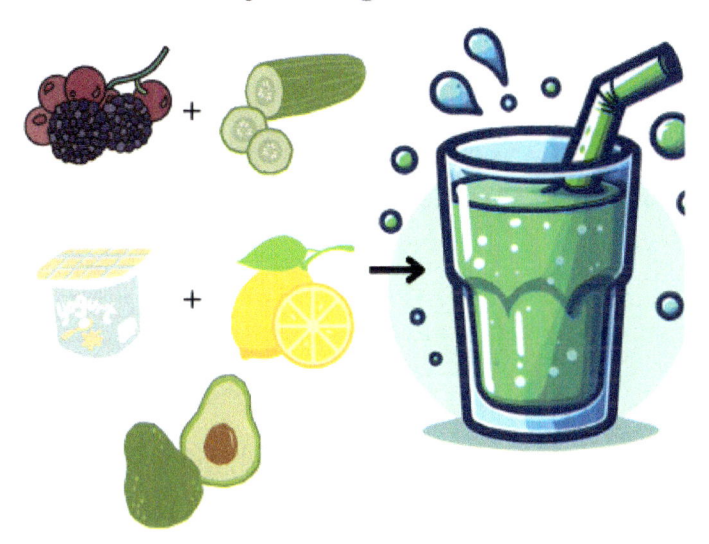

Ingredients:

- 1 cup blackberries
- 1/4 avocado
- 1/4 cup greek yogurt
- 1/2 cucumber
- 1/2 lemon

Underactive thyroids are becoming more of problem in our world. Cucumber provides a refreshing and hydrating base, while lemon adds a boost of vitamin C. Avocado contributes to high amounts of zinc to produce thyroid hormone production. Greek yogurt not only enhances the texture but also provides probiotics that can support gut health—a crucial aspect of thyroid regulation.

Bladder Health Boost

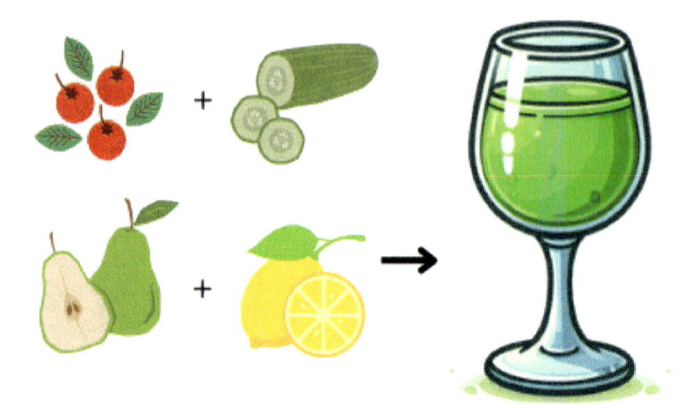

Ingredients:

- 1/2 cucumber
- 1/2 cup of cranberries
- 1/2 lemon
- 1 pear

Cucumber provides a hydrating and soothing foundation for this blend, promoting overall bladder health by ensuring proper hydration. Cranberries, renowned for their role in bladder health, work to prevent bacteria from adhering to the bladder walls, reducing the risk of urinary tract infections. Lemon enhances the vitamin C content, supporting the immune system and further fortifying bladder health. The pear prevents the formation of urinary tract stones, promoting a healthier and more comfortable urinary system.

Gum Disease Killer

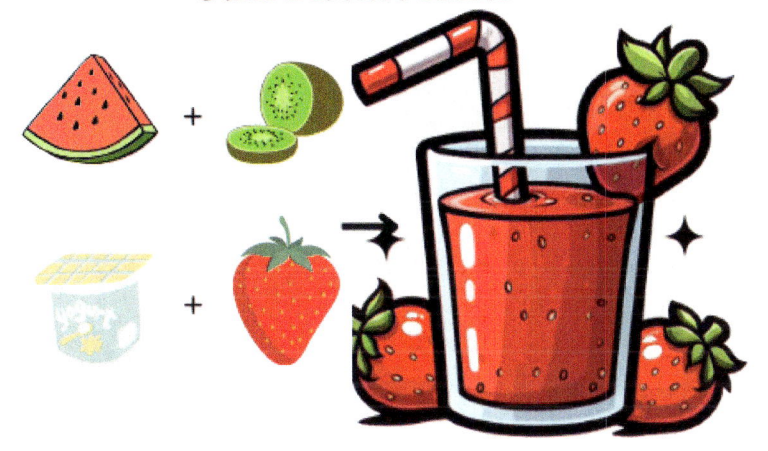

Ingredients:

- 1/2 cup strawberries
- 1/2 kiwi
- 1/2 cup watermelon
- 1/4 cup greek yogurt

Smelly breathe and gum disease are two things we don't need or want in our lives. Strawberries, known for their vitamin C content, provide crucial antioxidants that can help maintain gum health. Kiwi adds a delightful tartness and contributes additional vitamin C. Watermelon inhibits plaque buildup on your teeth. The inclusion of Greek yogurt not only enhances the texture but also introduces probiotics that may support oral microbiome balance—a vital aspect of gum health.

The Eye Visualiser

Ingredients:

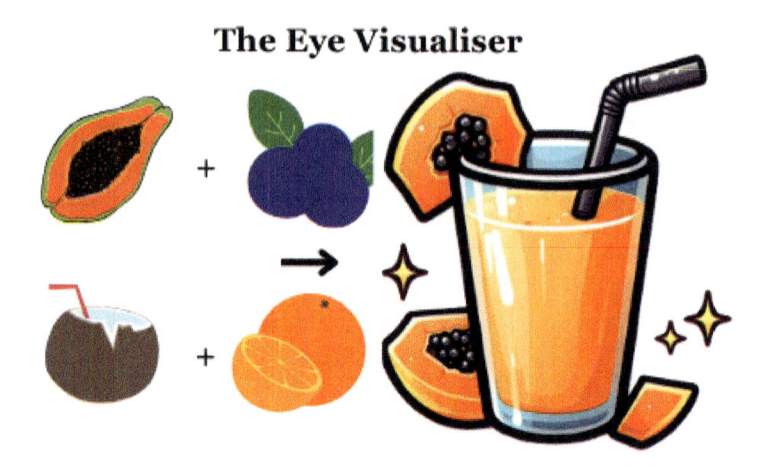

- 1/2 cup blueberries
- 1/2 cup orange
- 1/2 papaya
- 200ml coconut water

In my opinion, the eyes are by far the most important organ in our body as we perceive 80% of impressions through our eyes. Blueberries, renowned for their rich antioxidant content, provide vital nutrients that may help protect the eyes from oxidative stress and age-related conditions. Oranges contribute vitamin C, which supports the health of blood vessels in the eyes. The half a papaya provides beta-carotene, which is beneficial for maintaining good vision and protects our eyes from harmful blue light.

Pancreas Health

Ingredients:

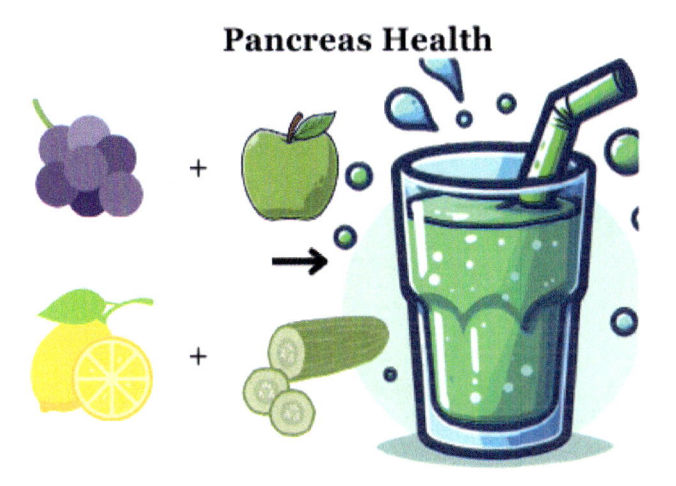

- 1/2 cucumber
- 1/2 green apple
- 1/2 lemon
- 1/2 cup red grapes

Your pancreas plays a pivotal role in the utilisation of sugar for energy following the process of digestion. In this healthful blend, cucumber forms a fundamental electrolyte base, assisting in the maintenance of essential bodily functions. The incorporation of a crisp green apple and red grapes not only adds fibre to the blend but also introduces resveratrol, a potent compound recognized for its impressive anti-inflammatory properties and its potential in combatting cancer.

Clean Colon Blend

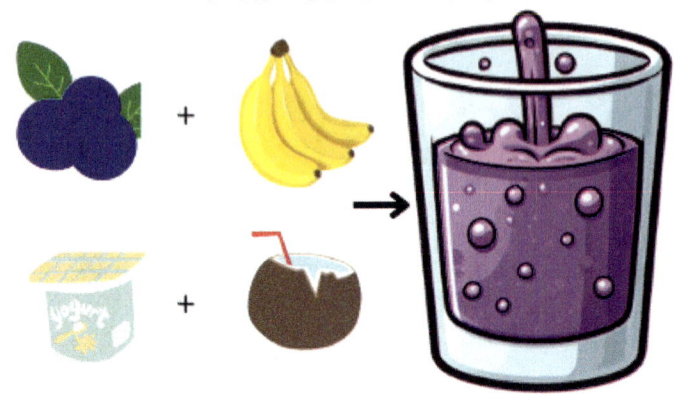

Ingredients:

- 1 cup blueberries
- 1 med-large banana
- 1/2 cup yogurt
- 150ml coconut water

If the colon is inflamed or damaged, the body can't absorb essential nutrients or get rid of waste efficiently. Blueberries, rich in antioxidants and dietary fiber, contribute to smoother digestion and help maintain a healthy colon. The banana adds additional dietary fiber, supporting regularity and optimal colon function. Yogurt introduces probiotics that balance your gut microbiome—a key aspect of colon health. Coconut water hydrates and replenishes electrolytes, aiding in overall digestive comfort.

Healthy Heart

Ingredients:

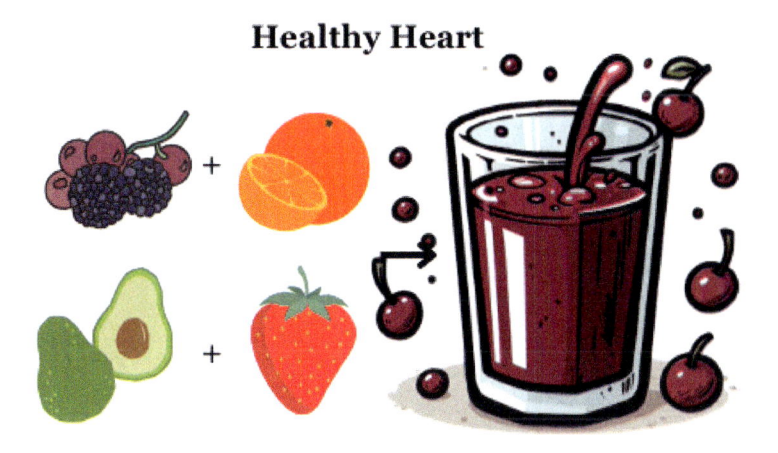

- 1/2 cup strawberries
- 1/2 cup blackberries
- 1 orange
- 1/2 avo

Heart health is crucial to our survival and pumping nutrient-rich blood throughout your body. The berry mix, packed with anthocyanins and fibre that support cardiovascular health. Oranges provide vitamin C, which may help improve heart function. The inclusion of an avocado introduces heart-healthy fats to reduce cholestrol levels.

Muscle Gainer Shake

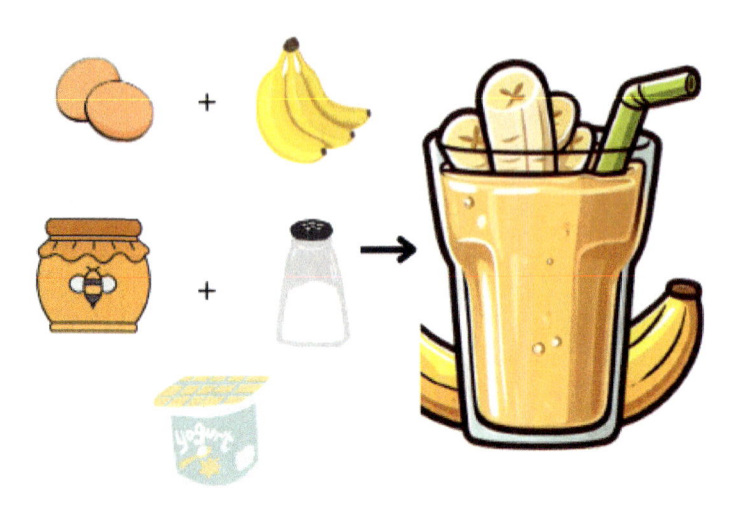

Ingredients:

- 5 egg whites
- 2 bananas
- 1 tbsp honey
- 2 tbsp yogurt
- 1/2 tsp salt

After each workout, it becomes crucial to replenish your body with the appropriate nutrients. This entails selecting foods that offer an adequate protein content while keeping fat levels relatively low and carbohydrate intake on the higher side. To achieve this post-workout nutritional balance, we can opt for a creative twist by incorporating fruits instead of relying solely on grains and potatoes.

Muscle Gainer Shake

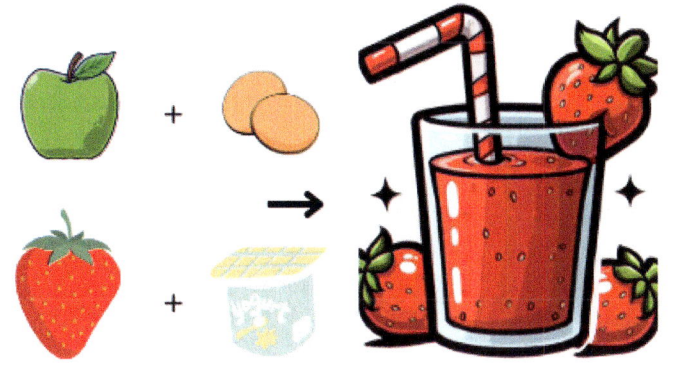

Ingredients:

- 5 egg whites
- 2 cups strawberries
- 2 tbsp yogurt
- 1 apple

Fruits offer a wealth of vitamins, minerals, and antioxidants that can aid in recovery, reduce muscle soreness, and support overall health. By making this subtle yet beneficial dietary adjustment, you can optimise your post-workout nutrition and promote your fitness journey's success, without the added toxicity from grains.

Muscle Gainer Shake

Ingredients:

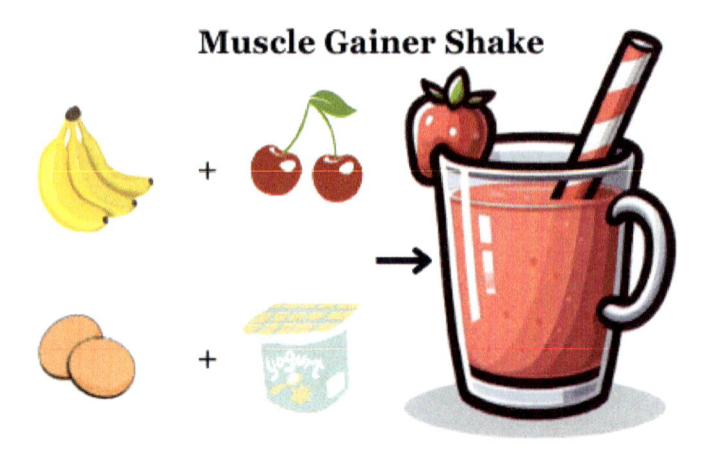

- 5 egg whites
- 2 bananas
- 1/2 cup cherries
- 2 tbsp yogurt

Incorporating fruits as part of your post-workout refueling strategy not only offers a delicious alternative but also provides valuable health benefits. The natural sugars in fruits, such as fructose and glucose, are easily absorbed by the body, making them an ideal choice for replenishing glycogen stores and kickstarting the recovery process.

Sex drive booster

Ingredients:

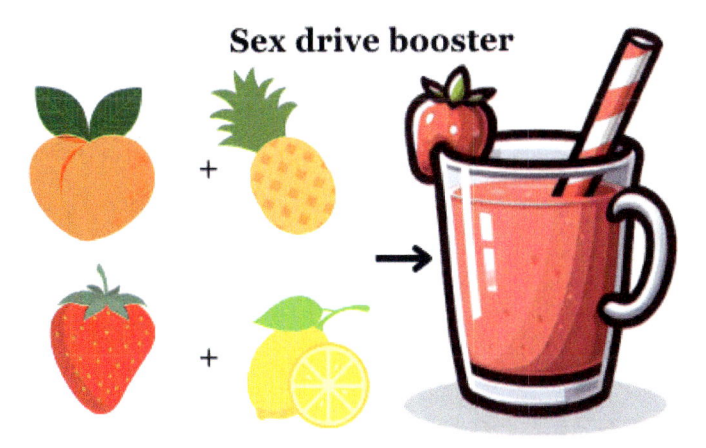

- 1/2 lemon
- 1 cup strawberries
- 1/4 pineapple
- 1 peach

The problem with testosterone going down is, men are starting to lose their sex drive because they are losing confidence and tend to struggle more now with performance issues. So skip the pills and have these drinks! This drink contains half a squeezed lemon, one cup of strawberries, a quarter of a pineapple and one peach. Peaches are high in vitamin C, which can improve sperm quality. The Thiamine in pineapple provides a surge of energy to the body too, thus increasing sexual stamina. Strawberries provide a boost in blood flow. lemon has been shown to increase blood flow aswell.

Sex drive booster

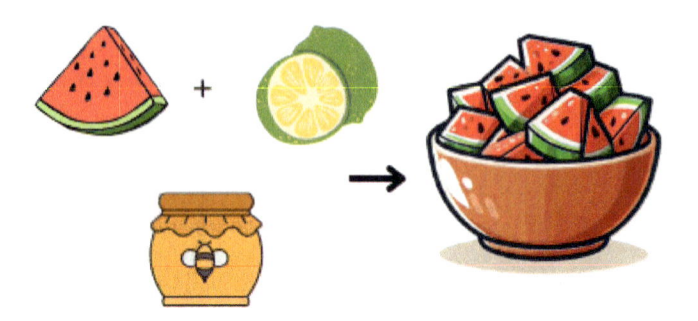

Ingredients:

- 1 tsp honey
- 1/4 watermelon
- 1/2 lime

This here is not a shake, its a snack you can have in a small bowl. It's super simple. Limes help to lower the levels of cortisol in your body. The minerals and enzymes in honey, increase blood flow to the genitals, which provides sustained energy and performance. Watermelon contains Citrulline, which is basically the natural viagra. It boosts arousal and increases blood flow.

Sex drive booster

Ingredients:

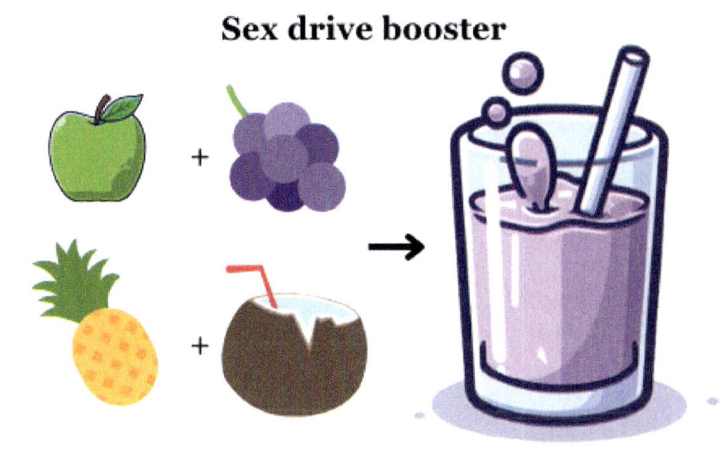

- 1/4 pineapple
- 1/2 cup grapes
- 200ml coconut water
- 1 apple

In one study, researchers linked a higher fruit intake to a 14 percent reduction in the risk of ED. Instead poisoning yourself with pills, rather have a juice packed with antioxidants and essential nutrients. Your body will thank you and so will your partner. The polyphenols from the grapes may improve the function of a woman's blood vessels, increasing blood flow to her nether regions. The coconut with those grapes will increase female natural lubrication as well. The pineapple contains bromelain, which can increase a man's sex desire by stimulating testosterone production. The apple increased blood flow.

Gut Health

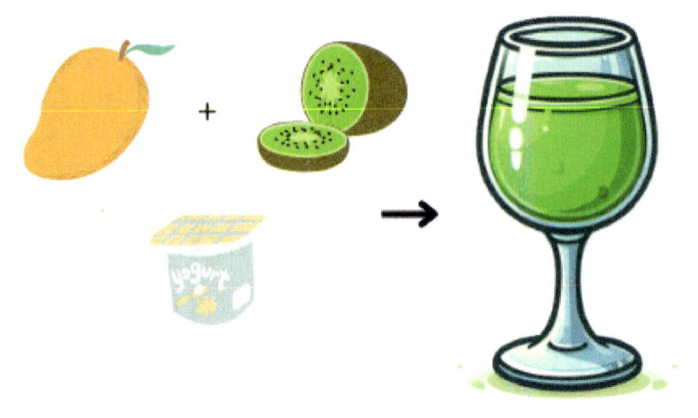

Ingredients:

- 1/2 mango
- 1 kiwi
- 3 tbsp yogurt

Ensuring a healthy gut is so important. If your gut is inflamed, you are prone to developing an autoimmune condition and even smelly breath. The mango aids the breakdown and digestion of protein, and also fibre, which facilitates smoother flow of food and wastes through the digestive tract. Kiwi eases bloating and reduces digestive discomfort. The microbes in yogurt can help support your gut and overall health.

Gallstone Prevention

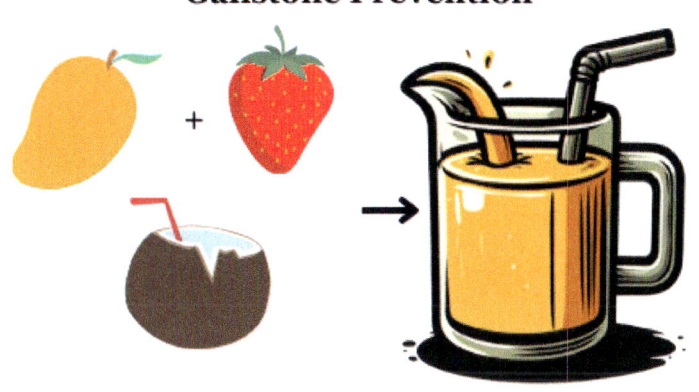

Ingredients:

- 1/2 mango
- 1/2 cup strawberries
- 250ml coconut water

Your gallbladder stores and secrete bile, which helps your body digest fats. When you develop gallstones, it blocks the flow of bile. If they are left untreated, it may increase your chance of gallbladder cancer and pancreatitis. So let's make a drink to help ease that pressure off. The mango helps in reducing the risk of gallstone formation. Strawberries are packed with antioxidants and Vitamin C. The coconut water is essential to stay hydrated with vital minerals.

Bone Fortifier

Ingredients:

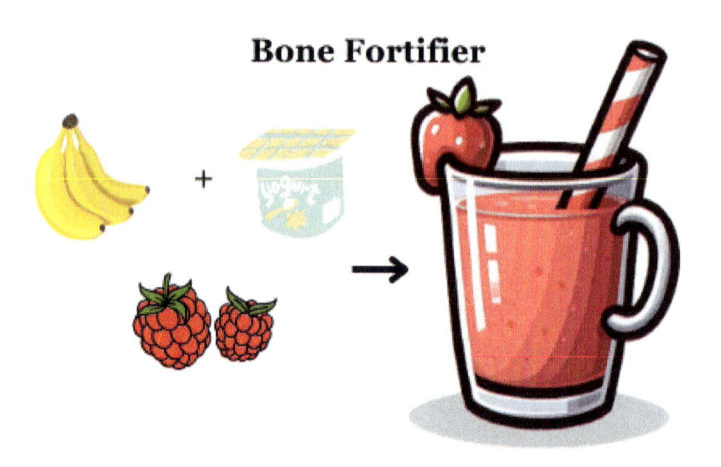

- 1 banana
- 1 cup yogurt
- 1/2 cup raspberries

Bones protect your brain, heart, and other organs from injury. Bones consist mainly of two minerals, calcium and collagen. You are gonna struggle getting calcium and collagen with plants only. So the combination of fruit and dairy content is perfect. This drink will consist of 1 banana, 1 cup of yogurt and half a cup of raspberries. The banana is packed with potassium, which helps boost the bone mineral density. The yogurt is packed with minerals, most importantly calcium, for bone strength. The raspberries are one the packed with ellagic acid which prevents calcium breakdown.

Hit the Hay

Ingredients:

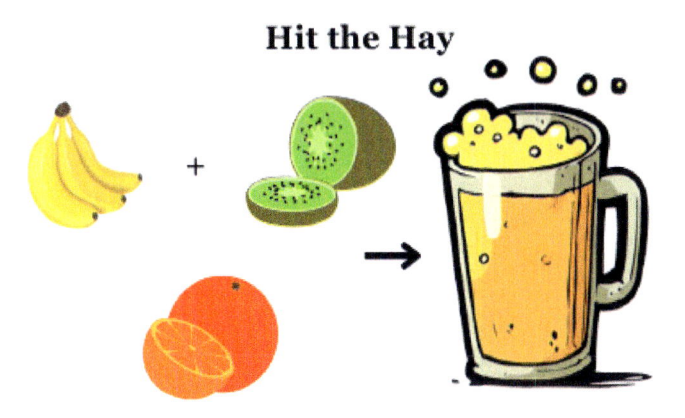

- 1 orange
- 1 banana
- 1 kiwi

Sleep improves your brain performance, mood, and health. If you do NOT get adequate sleep, the risk of contracting diseases and disorders are far higher. This drink will definitely help you fall asleep. The bananas contain serotonin, which is a precursor to melatonin and may help you to fall and stay asleep. Oranges aid in the synthesis of serotonin and dopamine. Kiwi contains serotonin, which help us relax and fall asleep.

PERSONAL CARE PRODUCTS

While we have scrutinised our diets and sought out healthier lifestyles, the role of personal care products in our overall health often goes unnoticed. These products, ranging from shampoos and lotions to cosmetics and fragrances, have become an integral part of our daily routines. Yet, what if I told you that these very items may harbour ingredients that have the potential to disrupt our hormonal balance, increase our risk of cancers, and contribute to a bunch of other health issues?

Personal care products are not subjected to the pre-market approval process by the FDA. This regulatory framework implies that companies are not obligated to demonstrate the safety or efficacy of these products before making them available to the public. Personal care products designed specifically to address or prevent health conditions fall under a different category. These products undergo a thorough safety processes by the FDA before they are granted the green light for commercial distribution.

It can be tricky to know if a product has risky stuff in it. You can try checking the label, but some chemicals have different names or abbreviations. And sometimes, they don't show up on the label at all, but they're still in there. So, it's a bit like playing detective when you're shopping.

Being mindful of avoiding harmful chemicals in your daily routines can contribute to your family's well-being. However, there are moments when you should exercise extra caution. Certain life stages can make people more susceptible to chemical exposure.

When looking out for personal care products, search up that product with the word "lawsuit" next to it on a private browser. This is just an effective method to see if that company is being sued for potential dangers.

Parabens are a group of chemicals widely used as artificial preservatives in cosmetic and body care products. Parabens are found in various skincare products, especially those with high water content like shampoos and conditioners that people use daily. They are effective against certain microbes. These chemicals are absorbed through the skin, processed by the body, and eliminated in urine and bile. Cosmetics often contain a mix of parabens, with methyl, ethyl, propyl, isopropyl, butyl, and isobutylparaben being the most common types. Parabens can mimic oestrogen in the body, disrupting hormone systems and impacting reproductive health, fertility, and birth outcomes. A 2016 UC Berkeley study discovered that even low levels of butylparaben, once considered safe, can activate cancer-related genes and promote breast cancer cell growth.

To lower your exposure to parabens, start by checking the ingredient list on the back of product labels. Watch out for ingredients ending in "paraben," like methylparaben, propylparaben, ethylparaben, butylparaben, isobutylparaben, and isopropylparaben, and steer clear of products containing them.

Parabens can be found in products across various price ranges, including high-end luxury beauty brands. Here are some examples of products that may contain parabens:

- Cerave hydrating facial wash.
- Lancome mascara
- Laura Mercier tinted moisturiser
- Chanel Vitalumier Aqua foundation
- Laura Mercier lip glace
- Laura Mercier Invisible Pressed setting powder
- Charlotte Tilbury eyeshadow

Talc is a mineral made up mainly of magnesium, silicon, and oxygen. As a powder, it absorbs moisture well and helps to stop friction, making it useful for keeping skin dry and helping prevent rashes. Talc finds extensive application in cosmetics like baby powder and adult body and facial powders, in addition to being a common ingredient in various other consumer goods. The problem with talc is that in a November 2020 study, found 14% of the talc-containing makeup tested also contained asbestos.

There has been speculation that the use of talcum powder could potentially be linked to ovarian cancer when applied to the genital area, with concerns that the powder particles might travel through the reproductive organs to the ovaries.

Numerous studies in women have explored this potential connection between talcum powder and ovarian cancer, but the findings have been inconclusive. Some studies have reported a slight increase in risk, while others have found no such increase.

You have alternative options to talc-based products that are natural and efficient at absorbing moisture while ensuring a fresh feeling. For instance, you can explore various uses of baking soda for your skin and hair.

Corn starch is another viable choice that can soothe skin irritations effectively. You can apply it to alleviate discomfort from bug bites, chafed skin, sunburns, jock itch, athlete's foot, and diaper rash.

Formaldehyde

Formaldehydec is a clear and smelly gas that can pose health risks if encountered by individuals at some point in their lives, with varying degrees of exposure among different people.

While you can craft an exceptional cleanser, moisturiser, or beauty product, the absence of a preservative could result in its limited shelf life, typically lasting only a few weeks. The introduction of formaldehyde-releasing agents into cosmetics initially aimed to prevent spoilage, guard against bacterial or fungal contamination, and extend their product lifespan.

The primary suspects within the beauty industry? Nail polishes and nail polish removers top the list as the most problematic. Additionally, hair products in general, along with baby shampoo and soap, may also contain formaldehyde or substances that release formaldehyde.

Here's a list of formaldehyde-releasing agents to be mindful of in skincare and cosmetic products. It's important to note that there are additional formaldehyde releasers utilized in industrial applications like plywood:

- Benzylhemiformal
- 2-bromo-2-nitropropane-1,3-diol
- 5-bromo-5-nitro-1,3-dioxane
- Diazolidinyl urea
- DMDM hydantoin
- Formaldehyde
- Glyoxal
- Imidazolidinyl urea
- Methenamine
- Paraformaldehyde
- Polyoxymethylene urea
- Sodium hydroxymethylglycinate
- Quaternium-15

Sunscreen products are meant for lifelong application so it's crucial for companies producing sunscreen ingredients and products to thoroughly assess their potential short-term and long-term health effects.

In 2021, the Food and Drug Administration (FDA), responsible for overseeing sunscreen safety, introduced updated regulations. Based on available information, it determined that only two ingredients, zinc oxide and titanium dioxide, could be deemed safe and effective.

However, twelve other ingredients lacked sufficient data and were not generally recognized as safe and effective. These ingredients included avobenzone, cinoxate, dioxybenzone, ensulizole, homosalate, meradimate, octinoxate, octisalate, octocrylene, oxybenzone, padimate O, and sulisobenzone. In 2021, the European Commission examined the safety of three organic ultraviolet (UV) filters: oxybenzone, homosalate, and octocrylene. It concluded that two of them were unsafe at current usage levels and proposed limiting their concentrations.

Studies published by the FDA revealed that ingredients like oxybenzone, octinoxate, octisalate, octocrylene, homosalate, and avobenzone are systemically absorbed after a single use and can live in the skin and bloodstream for weeks. Sunscreen ingredients have also been detected in breast milk, urine, and blood plasma samples. Continuous exposure to sunscreen chemicals raises concerns, particularly due to insufficient safety data for most ingredients. Oxybenzone has been associated with hormone disruption in numerous studies, amplifying concerns about its use.

CONCLUSION

When we prioritise our health, we are essentially investing in our future. We strive for optimal physical fitness, mental clarity, emotional resilience, and overall vitality. It's not just about the absence of illness; it's about embracing a lifestyle that enhances our physical strength, mental acuity, and emotional balance.

Much like a one-legged duck faces limitations, neglecting our health can impose restrictions on our ability to fully engage with life's opportunities and pleasures. Poor health can become a barrier to pursuing our passions, achieving our dreams, and enjoying the feeling of being alive.

I want to emphasise that this book is an introduction to a much broader journey. It has been my pleasure to share with you a glimpse of the vast landscape of resources available to empower us in our quest for a healthier, more informed life.

This is just the beginning. Each resource as well as common sense, discussed in these pages represents a treasure trove of knowledge, waiting to be delved into further. As I continue to study and learn every day, my aspiration is to delve deeper into these individual resources, exploring their intricacies and sharing more in-depth insights with you.

With the right knowledge and guidance, we can demystify the complexities of fitness, nutrition, and overcome the barriers that may have held us back in the past. The synergy of proper nutrition, well-being resources, and a sound fitness plan is the key to conquering the metabolic maze. It's a holistic approach that equips us to live our lives to the fullest, ensuring that we thrive not only in the present but for years to come

Joshua Bassett

Printed in Great Britain
by Amazon